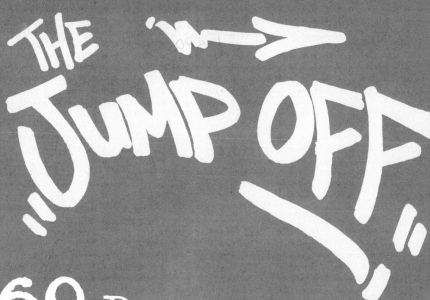

THE "JUMP OFF"

60 Days to a Hip-Hop Hard Body

MARK JENKINS

WITH JEFF O'CONNELL

HarperResource
An Imprint of HarperCollinsPublishers

DISCLAIMER

This book is written as a source of information only. The information contained in this book should by no means be considered a substitute for the advice of a qualified medical professional, who should always be consulted before beginning any new diet, exercise, or other health program.

All efforts have been made to ensure the accuracy of the information contained in this book as of the date published. The author and the publisher expressly disclaim responsibility for any adverse effects arising from the use or application of the information contained herein.

The availability of the downloadable music files from the Web site located at www.infitness.com/thejumpoff (the "Web Site") is referenced in this book solely for informational purposes. Such files are not a part of this book. The authors are solely responsible for the operation of, and the accessibility of downloadable music files from, the Web Site. In addition, the authors and the publisher expressly disclaim any liability for the failure to deliver the music files to a user from the Web Site, and any damage to a user's computer and related equipment and software resulting from the downloading of music from the Web Site.

HarperCollins books may be purchased for educational, business, or sales promotional use. For information, please write: Special Markets Department, HarperCollins Publishers Inc., 10 East 53rd Street, New York, NY 10022.

FIRST EDITION

Food styling and photography by Rick Schaff Productions © 2004.

Photograph on page 72 courtesy International Fitness © 2004.
Photographs on pages 73, 105, 118, and 181 courtesy AP/Wide World Photos.
Photograph on page 106 copyright © 2004 by Justin Jay.
All other photographs copyright © 2003 by Daven Baptiste.

INTERIOR DESIGN BY RENATO STANISIC

Library of Congress Cataloging-in-Publication Data

Jenkins, Mark, 1970–
    The jump off: 60 days to a hip-hop hard body/Mark Jenkins with Jeff O'Connell—1st ed.
        p.   cm.
    Includes index.
    ISBN 0-06-058818-7
        1. Physical fitness.   2. Exercise.   3. Health.   I. Title: 60 days to a hip-hop hard body.
        II. Title: Sixty days to a hip-hop hard body.   III. O'Connell, Jeff, 1963–   IV. Title.

GV481.J455   2005
613.7—dc22   2004047304

05 06 07 08 09 ❖ / RRD 10 9 8 7 6 5 4 3 2 1

I DEDICATE THIS BOOK TO ALL THE PEOPLE OUT THERE WHO HAVE STRUGGLED WITH THEIR WEIGHT.
DON'T GIVE UP!

IT'S ONLY A MATTER OF TIME AS LONG AS YOU
KEEP TRYING.

I ALSO WANT TO DEDICATE <u>THE JUMP OFF</u> TO MY SON, LEE.
I LOVE YOU VERY MUCH!

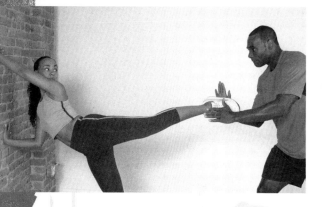

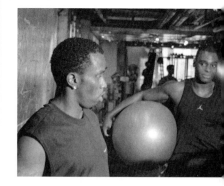
EXCLUSIVE MUSIC OFFER:

Go to www.infitness.com/TheJumpOff to download a collection of original hip-hop compiled by the author to drive the pace of your workout session.

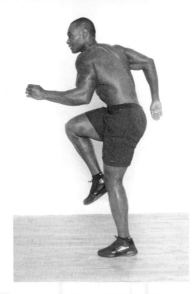

PART 3

THE FITNESS LIFESTYLE

CELEBRITY SIDEBARS

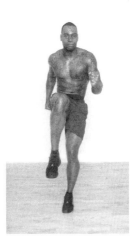

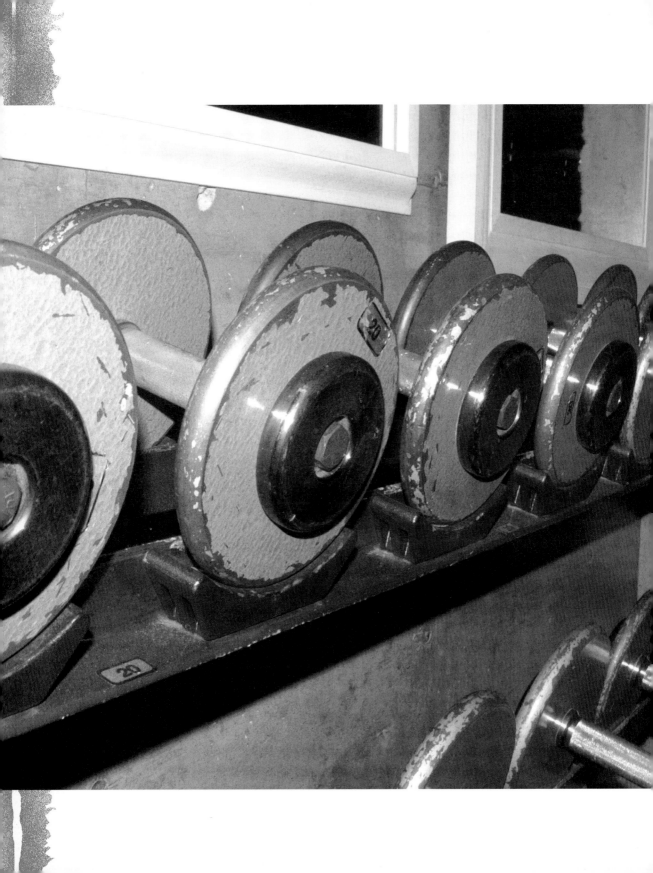

ACKNOWLEDGMENTS

I would like to say thanks to my editors Nick Darrell and Megan Newman, who were very patient and cool to deal with. Thanks to my man Jeff O'Connell, who cowrote this book with me. Thanks to Daven Baptiste for lacing the photos. Thank you to Tiffany Mossy, who was the female victim in *The Jump Off.* Also a big thank you to all my clients. You guys really put out and always make me proud. I have learned so much about strength, perseverance, and dedication from each and every one of you! Finally, I would like to thank my wife for all her love and support.

NATASHA, I LOVE YOU!

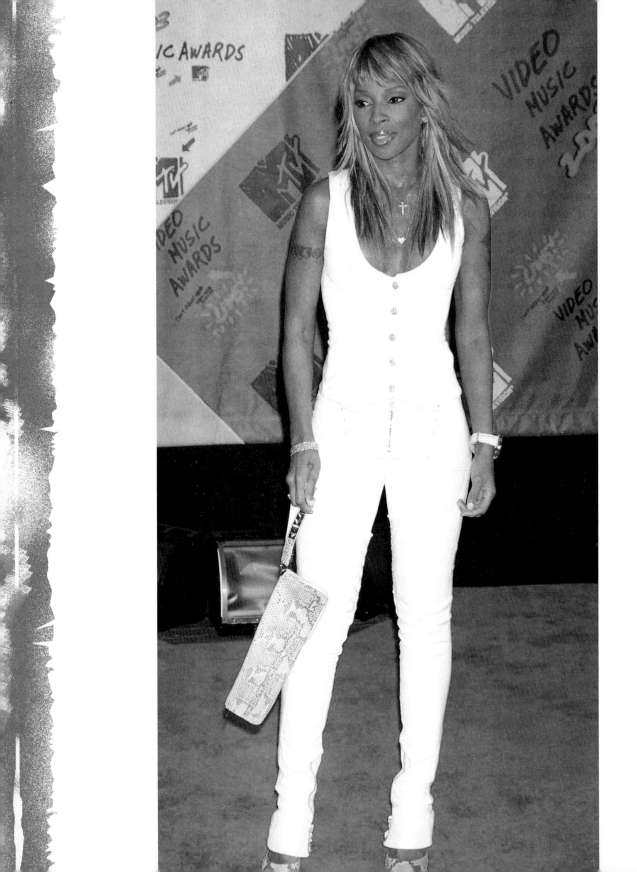

FOREWORD by Mary J. Blige

It was early 2002, and I was getting ready to hit the road in support of my CD *No More Drama*. It was my most highly anticipated tour ever, and along with that anticipation came major expectations. After all, the single "Family Affair" had already been No. 1, and the title track was now flying up the charts right behind it. The CD had also been nominated for a Grammy—Best R&B Album—and "Family Affair" had been nominated in the category of Best R&B Vocal Performance/Female.

Along with the excitement surrounding a new tour comes incredible amounts of pressure. It's that delicate balancing act almost all successful recording artists eventually have to make: nurturing your artistry and at the same time gearing up for something as logistically complicated as preparing a small army for battle. Add to that the incredible media demands that are placed on us today, and no wonder even the strongest artists often exhaust themselves on the road, mentally and physically—sometimes before the tour even starts!

This time, though, I had a secret weapon in my corner: Mark Jenkins. I had been training with Mark for the month leading up to opening night, and amazing things had been happening to my body. It was ironic and wonderful that he had come into my life just as *No More Drama* was blowing up, because that describes his approach to a T. He strips out all the BS and gets you to focus on exactly what you need to do to take control over your body, which is to exercise and eat right. And it all came together for me the night of the first show. A half hour or so before the curtain was to rise, I looked at myself in the mirror, and suddenly I was really buggin' off of the muscle popping out from my stomach and in my arms. With Mark's help, I had reached a goal I had never achieved before, and as a result I stepped on stage that night happy and brimming with confidence. If you saw any of those shows, you saw how the band and me tore it up.

I had tried to get in shape before, but for whatever reason, it hadn't worked out. By the time I hooked up with Mark, I was out of shape and overweight. I wasn't nearly as strong as I am right now, and that's because I had never trained *his* way before. His way isn't easy, believe me. Mark doesn't treat you with kid gloves. His approach woke up a lot of muscles that I didn't know existed, and he was constantly telling me to diet hard, *diet hard*, diet hard. It wasn't like I was depriving myself, though. I was actually eating six times a day. I was just eating differently.

It didn't happen overnight—I have to be truthful and honest—and for the first few weeks I didn't even really look at my body or pay attention, probably because I never used to like what I saw. But when I looked in the mirror that night at the show, I noticed some amazing things happening.

In essence, this book was my blueprint. You're holding all of the information that I, Puffy, and other recording artists have paid a lot of money to acquire, but only you can make the time to use this information. If you don't think you have the time, compare your schedule to mine or another superstar's and ask yourself again what your excuse is. Training was hard for me at first too, but now it's just like breathing. I like that analogy because training is something I do to keep my health up. This is not just a vanity thing for me anymore. The instructions Mark gives you aren't just to make muscles pop out of your stomach, it's so you can live a longer, healthier life.

Working out with Mark as your guide will enrich your life in so many ways. I know for a fact that the focus and discipline I've learned from Mark have made me a better artist. The connections are obvious to me only in hindsight: a lot of things you want to eat, you can't eat; a lot of the things you want to do a day or two before you go onstage, you can't do; and so on. It's all the same mind-set. Eventually, these small sacrifices won't require the same discipline they did initially. You'll live that way because when you're in better shape, you're happier. Working out really helps you to have a better day.

It's not going to happen overnight, and in the meantime, don't beat yourself up about your body. What you can't do right now, you can't do. But put your faith in *The Jump Off* and you'll be amazed at how quickly you transform your body, and how that transformation will improve your entire life. I'm living proof of the difference the Mark Jenkins approach can make.

—Mary J. Blige
July 2004

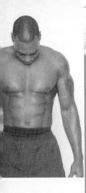
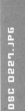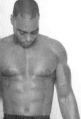
GETTING STARTED 1

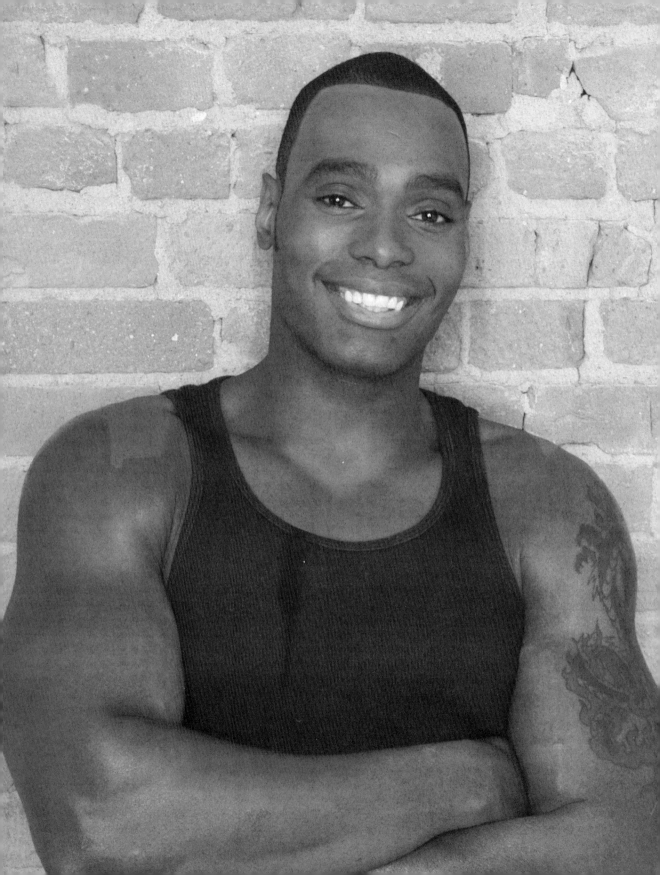

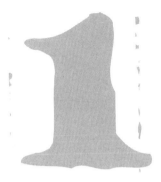

My Story

As I cruise through the Mediterranean Sea
on board P. Diddy's yacht, water as far as the eye
can see, I can't help but smile. The boat is
unbelievably tricked out, with rooms fit for kings.
The crew treats us like royalty too, anticipating
and attending to our every need. Best of all for
fitness fanatics like me, a cook prepares food for us
that tastes like it was reeled in 10 minutes ago. On
top of that, the gym is off the hook! I can't get over
my good fortune. I have the best gig in the world.

Can you believe I'm here **working?** That's right.
My name is Mark Jenkins, and I'm traveling in style
with one of my clients, P. Diddy. He needs to keep

training during R&R because in less than a month, he and I will have taken on the New York City Marathon to benefit kids in the New York public school system. The marathon is no joke, believe me. By the time he's finished, P. Diddy, a modern-day icon of style, will have lost five toenails in pursuit of this goal.

If you're thinking, "*If I had Diddy's bank account, I'd be in shape, too,*" then think again. No one has handed that guy anything; he's earned every dime of it by rolling his sleeves up and working incredibly hard for a very long time. In fact, free time, the one resource you need the most to get in shape, is the one thing that he has virtually none of, since he runs several multimillion-dollar empires simultaneously. The guy sleeps only four hours a night. Sometimes he's ready to train at three o'clock in the morning. I've even had to send him home because if he's too tired, it's a waste. Puffy really trains his butt off, and as you'll soon find out, I expect no less from you. That's the kind of attitude that you'll need to get in shape.

When I'm training Diddy or Mary J. Blige, I admit, I can't always believe it's for real. If a psychic had told me when I was a kid that I'd end up training those two superstars, I'd never have believed her. And they're just the latest in a long list of elite clients I've whipped into the best shape of their lives—Diddy, Mary, D'Angelo, Beyonce, LL Cool J, and Missy Elliott among them.

My current situation is a far cry from where I started out. I grew up in the Crown Heights Brooklyn, which was a tough place back in the early 1980s. My street was a refuge in a bad neighborhood, where gunshots rang out nightly. Our block was safer than the ones around it because the Brooklyn Botanic Gardens, the Brooklyn Museum, and the main branch of the Brooklyn Public

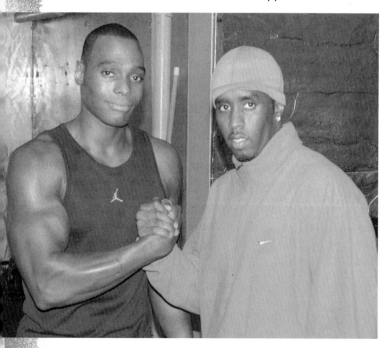

Me and Diddy arm wrestling.

Library were across the street and there were always police stationed nearby.

I remember days when my friends and I walked with screwdrivers in our pockets just to get to the YMCA to play ball. You had to pass through some dangerous neighborhoods on your way, and we wanted to be able to protect ourselves in case we got jumped. In high school I saw kids walking home barefoot through the snow after getting their sneakers stolen off their feet. When I'd reach my block, I'd stop for a second and let out a sigh of relief. It was so ill growing up back then, but that's just how it was. A lot of the guys I went to high school with are either in jail or dead.

My father died when I was 2, which didn't start things off in my favor. My mom remarried a man who was a former bodybuilder, so I guess you can say he made me body-conscious at an early age. Still, I didn't have a great relationship with him. He was a stepfather, which creates its own set of problems, but he was also an alcoholic and a strict disciplinarian, so we never did the typical father-son bonding things.

My mom didn't know what to do with me, so she started hauling me off to dancing school along with my older sister. For over six years I danced my butt off: tap, jazz, ballet, modern, along with some gymnastics. I even attended a junior high school for gifted kids with dancing as my talent. But when I hit puberty and started getting teased about dancing—being called a faggot and a sissy by my stepfather didn't help—I conformed by quitting. I transferred to a public junior high school and got introduced to other fine arts, like drinking and profanity.

That's when I started to put on weight. My mom is from Antigua and my stepfather is from Barbados, so the West Indian diet was the norm in our family. If you're not familiar with this diet, let me tell you, the starches will kill you. On top of that I would eat tons of candy, drink a gallon of milk a day, or down over half a pound of pasta in one sitting. It seemed like I was always hungry. The combination of lots of carbohydrate and very little activity was a recipe for disaster. My energy level went up and down like a roller coaster. I was running on sugar, which seriously impaired my ability to learn and stay focused.

I think I was overcompensating with food to make myself feel better about my home life and general insecurities. Dancing helped keep the weight off, but once I stopped, I didn't have another activity to replace it. By the time I hit high school, I had a 40-inch waist and my friends started calling me "Suck in the Gut" because I was always trying to disguise it. My self-esteem was a mess, and the challenges I faced at home weren't making it any easier.

When I was 17, my home life reached a critical point. For some time my mother had tolerated my rebelliousness, but she was less willing to indulge me as the years passed. One day she said, "If you don't want to listen to what I have to say, then get the hell out of my house." My mother had bankrupted herself to send my sister to Penn State University, and there was no dough left for me to go to college, even though I was doing okay academically. I figured I'd join the military. I thought it could offer me opportunities I wouldn't find in Crown Heights. Also, I wanted to get back in shape. After thorough research, I chose the Navy because it offered the most opportunities to travel and had the easiest boot camp.

From the minute I stepped off the bus that first day in 1988, I thought, *This is a mistake.* My stepfather was nothing compared to the drill sergeants who abused me from the start. I broke down in tears immediately—I was such a mama's boy. I'd never washed my own clothes or made my own bed before. No discipline! Even after weeks of training, I could barely run 2 miles or grunt out 20 push-ups. Luckily, a friend of mine named Keith Dorsette, who was a Marine, would run with me. Even though I never finished a run, I never would have made it through boot camp if he hadn't helped me train. (Thanks, Keith.) It got me used to moving again after having given up dancing. This was the first physical activity I had done in years, and I was only 17.

On the one hand, I wondered what I'd been thinking, placing myself in such a brutal environment. But on the other hand, I knew this experience was going to make a man out of me. Anyway, what did I have to lose? I could always go back to my mom's house, right? I figured I might as well stick it out, make the best of it, and learn from it.

The Navy's harsh regimen was a shock, but it taught me things that school didn't, like using your mind to overcome challenges. Physical failure can be tolerated in the military, but mental failure never is. It's one thing to give up because you can't go anymore, but it's a different thing to quit because you're tired of trying. *That's* failure. This philosophy applies to working out and to life in general. That's why I'm a huge advocate of tough love, and I'm going to give you a heavy dose of it throughout this book. Sometimes you need someone to ride you to get you to take action.

If you find these workouts demanding, the Navy's workouts were so intense

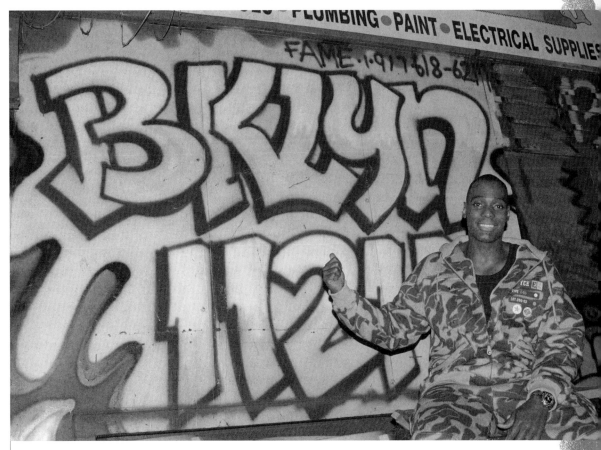

PLUMBING • PAINT • ELECTRICAL SUPPLIES
FAME • 1 • 917 618-62

Repping my boro!

that most of the guys couldn't finish them no matter what kind of shape they were in. The drills were made to break you and force you to fight as long and as hard as you could without quitting. You'll find this quality in the workouts that you're about to start. I ran drills until I fell to the ground and threw up. Then I'd get up and keep on running. I turned it into a mental challenge. *I will not let them break me,* I kept repeating to myself. *Brooklyn is tougher than this.* That got me through eight weeks of boot camp and the day I graduated was one of the proudest of my life.

After boot camp I was stationed in Fresno, California, as part of an F-18 squadron. One day, at the gym on base, I walked up to a group of the biggest guys in there and said, "Hey, I want to look like you guys. Can I train with you?" I'd lost

30 to 40 pounds in boot camp, but I still looked like a smaller version of Suck in the Gut—flabby and practically in need of a training bra. The guys stared at me, laughed, and asked, "Why should we train with you?" I told them that I'd train hard and I wouldn't quit, which must have been the right answer, because before I knew it we were rockin'. I didn't realize when I approached these guys that their idea of a spotting for a weight-lifting session mostly meant getting a slap on the back of the neck accompanied by, "Get that weight up!" I didn't mind, though, because I was starting to put together the whole fitness puzzle, lifting and cardio. My buddies pounded me on the weights, and I started getting bigger and bigger. After almost two years of lifting with them, I had 22-inch arms, 32-inch-thick legs and a 29-inch waist at 250 pounds. If anything, I think I overdid it!

Just as I was enjoying my newfound physique, the Gulf War broke out. I was planning on going to college, but the Gulf War broke out. I thought I was going to flex on the beach and get a lot of girls, *but the Gulf War broke out!* Next thing you know, I'm floating on a ship in the middle of the Indian Ocean with 5,000 other men and women, with a gas mask dangling from my belt. A slight change of plans.

Although I was still only 19, I matured fast because the circumstances got serious real quick. I started to contemplate what I wanted to do with the rest of my life. *What am I doing out here?* I thought. *What causes am I interested in putting my life on the line for?* Being on the ship, I found myself around veterans who had been in wars before. Here I was walking around like a tough guy, and these guys had actually seen combat. They were like, "You don't know jack! You're straight out of boot camp." But I *had* seen combat—on the streets of Brooklyn.

My cultural and social horizons expanded as well as my geographical ones. In high school I couldn't even speak to a girl, but now girls were approaching me whenever we'd reach port. You played as hard as you could on shore because in the back of your mind, you were thinking, *Man, I could die out here.* In addition to the general perils of war, working on an aircraft carrier is one of the most dangerous jobs in the world because there are so many ways you can get killed. One time I was securing some gear on deck, a plane flew by, and the sonic boom almost knocked me off the ship. I was hanging maybe 20 stories high over the ocean and nobody was there to pull me up. Luckily, I was in shape and was able to pull myself up. Otherwise I wouldn't be writing this book now.

Fortunately the aircraft carrier I was on during the war was equipped with two gyms, both situated under the catapults. It could be 100-plus degrees inside at any given time. Two gyms, 5,000 people—they were so crowded that it felt like jail. Planes were landing right above us, so the boat was rocking while we were squatting, benching, and lunging. Condensation from the catapults covered the floor, making it slippery. Everybody was training in steel-toed flight deck boots. It was very hard-core—and I loved it.

You really had to want it to train in those conditions after 12 hours on duty, but I never missed a workout. Workouts became my way to stay sane in an alien environment. I sent away for all the bodybuilding books and magazines and supplements I could get. I had nothing else to buy with my paycheck on the ship anyway. Being in a war is obviously very stressful, and working out was one of the few things that kept my spirits up and my energy level high.

In fact, I trained my first unofficial client on that aircraft carrier. One of my shipmates was so overweight that his body fat was nearing the threshold for getting the boot. Once you get too fat, you're not fighting fit, and they don't want you in there. I had been in that situation two years earlier, so I knew this guy could get in shape. He just needed good information and some hard-core motivation. So I started to work him out, making him train, diet, jump rope in his flight deck boots.

Eventually he achieved such good shape that I started getting a reputation on board as someone the other guys could turn to if they weren't happy with the way they looked and felt and wanted to take charge of the situation. So I trained them, too. I wasn't making any money at it, and I was shortchanging myself on sleep, but I found it so rewarding that I didn't mind, and it was fun. That was another thing I learned early on—that I would rather train than sleep.

It also made me feel better about the situation on the ship by taking my mind off the reality of why I was really there. Looking back, I actually think that my being a 19-year-old from Brooklyn worked to my advantage. I had seen people getting shot and thrown out of third-story windows before, whereas a lot of those more sheltered guys were really losing it out there. Guys would drink Scope and Listerine just to get by. One time I cleaned out a bathroom and found a crack pipe in there— on a Navy vessel with nuclear warheads! Guys did what they needed to do to deal with the stress, positive or negative, and sometimes they just cracked up.

So guess what? In 1992, after the Gulf War, I left the Navy. I moved back to New York and lived with my mom for a while. That drove me crazy, because she

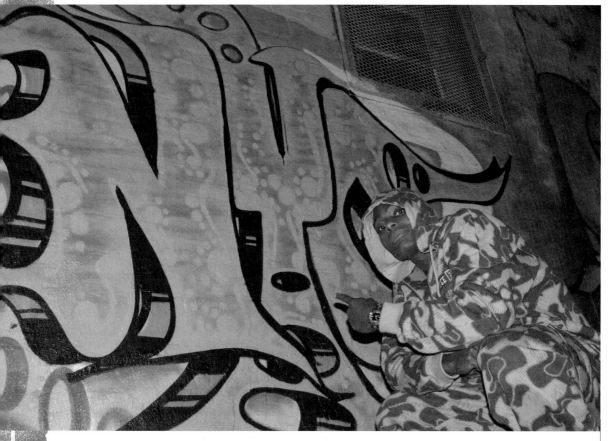

Where it all started.

still looked at me as the same wet-behind-the-ears kid I was before I'd left, not the man I'd become. She also kept checking my vitamins to see if they were steroids. All I was using was a Cybergenics workout kit and Joe Weider's Mega Mass 3000 weight-gain powder. That was my stack. That's all they really had back in the early days of supplements, and it taught me an important lesson that I'll pass on to you now: No matter what supplements you have, you still have to push it in the gym to make it happen.

So I moved out and got a job as a temp at a post office in Brooklyn. I hated the job and the hours (midnight to 8:30 A.M., five days a week), but after work I'd head straight to the gym. By then I was 250 pounds and rock solid, and I wanted to keep it that way. As much as I hated my job, I had enough discipline to stay with it until I found something else. It's not enough just to perform during the good times, when you're happy doing something. Sometimes you've got to show up every day just in order to create a better situation for yourself in the future. So one day in 1993, the gym manager who I always complained to about my terrible job and terrible hours finally offered me a gig. He said, "Mark, you're a good motivator. Why don't you get certified and work in the gym?" That's all I needed to hear. The next day I quit the post office job.

Something told me this was going to be a life-changing opportunity. Even though I was paid less than I was at the post office—maybe $5 an hour, plus $15 an hour for a private training session—it was well worth it. I wasn't just a spoke in the wheel anymore. I was doing something I liked, and I was really good at it. I could set my own hours, get my own clients, and be an entrepreneur. I felt like my individual strengths could shine through, because it was a one-on-one job.

Soon I was certified and became a personal trainer at a gym right across from Motown Records. One day one of my clients asked me if I could train Brandy, the young R&B singer who was slated to star in the TV sitcom *Moesha* and needed to get into shape. I was like, "How do you know Brandy?"

"I'm Brandy's publicist," she said.

I could have kicked myself for not having asked her what she did till then. At that moment, I made a note to myself: Ask clients what they do for a living, Dummy. I agreed to train Brandy but had no idea how much to charge. Finally we agreed on $70 an hour. For a guy now living in the projects of Fort Greene, Brooklyn, it seemed like I had hit the lotto. I thought I was going to be rich, but I trained with Brandy for only two weeks before she flew off to California. I could see a bag of money with wings flying away with her.

It was tough to see that opportunity go, but for the first time I started to see training as a way of really making it. I imagined that if I could book eight to ten clients at $70 an hour, I'd be making $700 a day! I could generate a lot of money and perhaps start my own business, maybe even open my own gym. I also thought about targeting black artists and celebrities, with the idea that I could maybe teach and inspire black youth through the example of these artists. It dawned on me that I could really make a positive impact and make money at the same time. I got to be a leader again, trying to help all these people get in shape—many of whom were in the same situation I was in before I got it together in the military. I could use my hard-core military training style on some unsuspecting civilians.

The disparities between black people and white people became even clearer to me in the workforce. One key difference was fitness. Only a few blacks had memberships at the Vertical Club where I worked. In 1993, black people and fitness wasn't really happening. Some of the first people I approached with the idea laughed. *Black people working out? Payin' money for that? Nobody's feelin' that. They're not going to pay you to do that.* Even my closest friends asked me how I planned to pull all this off. I was just one trainer in a crowded city with thousands of trainers in thousands of gyms. But I didn't let that reality stop me. One of them had to be the best, I figured—might as well be me. Nobody's going to work as hard, I thought, so I definitely have a shot. My past victories gave me the courage and the hunger to really want it and go after it.

Besides, I had another key asset that a lot of other trainers didn't. I'd battled my own weight issues in the past, and still do. I really knew what to say because I knew what I had needed to hear sometimes. I didn't look like Suck in the Gut anymore, but I always felt like he was right around the corner. I knew I could strongly motivate and inspire my clients because I was still fighting this battle every day. I'm in the trenches with them today, still.

What I needed was a plan. I asked my successful clients for advice, and that's when I started to realize that most successful people have the same habits. My clients where like, "Mark, you need a publicist!" But when I pointed out that I was living in the projects with no money, they would tell me, "Well, train a publicist." So I found a publicist and I trained him. I would train a photographer to get free pictures, and train an intern here and there in hopes of getting closer to a higher-up who might be connected to a celebrity. I also started training CEOs in exchange for free lunches, during which I would take notes on the advice they would lay on me: Be smart and stand firm in negotiations. Be the best, and then charge like you're the best. Train people for free when you want to barter, but always stand firm on your prices. Master your craft and make it work for you.

This went on for years, and because I was the king of freebies, I even had to take on another job, bouncing in clubs at night. But I knew that if I had faith and continued going 100 percent, something had to give. I couldn't see the next opportunity, but I kept on going, knowing it was just around the corner.

In 1999, after seven years of patience and hard work, my big break arrived. I got the invitation to train D'Angelo after training his publicist, and I knew it was time. I informed his people that they would need to pay for one month in advance at $100 per session. At first they said the price was too steep for a trainer, but I convinced them that not only would D'Angelo get in fantastic shape, but he would also set a precedent in music as the best-conditioned artist of his generation. Sold! They advanced me my money, and I immediately quit my job and started my own training company, knowing I would have to dedicate myself completely to getting him into shape. I camped out in front of his hotel room and I followed him to the studio, training his mind as well as his body. D'Angelo is usually late for sessions, so I had to learn to crash wherever he was supposed to be and just wait. I knew that if he got into peak condition, it would really be huge for both of us.

I made fitness important to him by making it important to everybody around him. This was key to his success. I trained his assistants so that they would buy into what I was doing with D, rather than criticizing or otherwise undercutting the things we were trying to achieve. The end result could not have been better— with 5 percent body fat and perfect muscular symmetry, he performed his video *Untitled* topless. Based to a large extent of the buzz created by that video, his CD sales went through the roof. Finally, I could see it happening—all because I persevered when it wasn't happening.

I got some pub for D'Angelo's transformation, but I didn't let up on my freebie training sessions. They were a winning strategy that eventually hooked me up with my next big client. My barber, who I was training for free, turned me onto another of his clients who worked for Mary J. Blige. My barber told him, "Yo, this is the guy, the trainer who did D." He was like, "Yo, you gotta get Mary. She's going on tour. Come to the studio tonight, and if Mary likes you, it's on." She saw I was serious about getting her in shape and put me on her team. In two months I helped her drop 40 pounds.

My strategy was starting to pay off. Little did I know that while following Mary J. Blige on her next tour, I was to meet my soul mate and future wife, Natasha. Unfortunately, I was still depressed over a recent breakup, and I couldn't get into the social scene the way I had planned to. Natasha approached me one night to ask what was wrong, and I told her about my struggle.

A few days later, Natasha was out on a date with someone else (she says it wasn't a date) and I rode up on a Harley I had rented. She was about 100 yards away, so I revved the engine and she looked over. At that moment I knew we had made a connection.

Finally we made a pact: If we were still in love by the time Mary's concert tour hit Vegas, we would get married. Three weeks later the bus pulled into Vegas and we got married, after only six weeks of knowing each other. After that, everything hit an all-time high. Her ability to handle the business side of things allowed me to focus on transforming my clients in the shortest amount of time possible. By this point I'd made a name for myself by transforming more and more people, like LL Cool J and Johnnie Cochran, just to name a few.

Eventually, P. Diddy heard about me and wanted to put me on his team. This was one of the biggest challenges in my life, because I knew this guy wasn't used to taking orders. But I figured that if we got him into a competitive setting, he would rise to the occasion, thus getting himself into peak condition. He stepped up big time, and, at my urging, we eventually ran the New York City Marathon together. While the average person takes eight months to a year to get ready for a marathon, we did it in eight weeks. He also got everybody on board and turned it into something bigger than I could ever have imagined. We ran for the public school system. How cool was this: training P. Diddy *and* running for charity?

Natasha was doing her thing for the business, too. In 2003, she secured deals for this book, a DVD, and a supplement kit. Inside the latter were a diet booklet and my workout video, allowing you to experience a training session with me first-hand, just like my celebrity clients did. The name of the kit is *Work It,* and I have to admit, I'm proud that it brought dietary supplements to a new market. It's the first time a supplement box has featured a black man who actually has a stake in the product. I was breaking barriers as well.

In the latter half of 2003, the *Work It* kit went nationwide, and I still can't believe I have my supplements in every GNC store in America. I'm on the box, so people of color can identify. The African American and Latino audiences need physical fitness, especially because of the way it boosts self-esteem. There are more obese kids of color out there than ever, and believe me, it affects their self-image. I want to give these kids the gift that I got and watch it transform their lives the way it transformed mine and those of my clients.

I wanted to be a civil rights activist when I grew up, and in a sense, I've been able to do a lot of good using fitness as my pulpit. When I started, I didn't know how successful I'd become; I just had faith and attacked whatever I was doing at 100 percent, even when it was just working in the post office or bar bouncing. As a result, now I'm able to get these hip-hop hard-bodies to look the way they do in videos and movies, and millions of young people copy their heroes. The artists pull in the audience through their talent, and my handiwork inspires fans to adopt a fit, healthy lifestyle—a killer combination.

Once I got myself in shape, I felt I could exert more control over the world around me, in all its manifestations: business, family, and so on. That's what I hope you get from *The Jump Off*—not only a kick-ass workout, but also inspiration and faith in your own power to better yourself.

After all, faith is what brought me to where I am today—faith and a willingness to believe in my personal vision, stick with it and not be afraid to see things outside the box. If I hadn't pushed myself and believed in myself along the way, I wouldn't be in this unbelievable place—training with Puffy, running 20 miles with Alberto Salazar, checking Calvin Klein's refrigerator to offer advice on how he can improve his eating habits, and living happily married to my soul mate with our brand-new daughter.

So the Jump Off is just what the name implies—a beginning, a start. It's a 60-day program for achieving a hip-hop hard body and the start of a journey that can change the rest of your life.

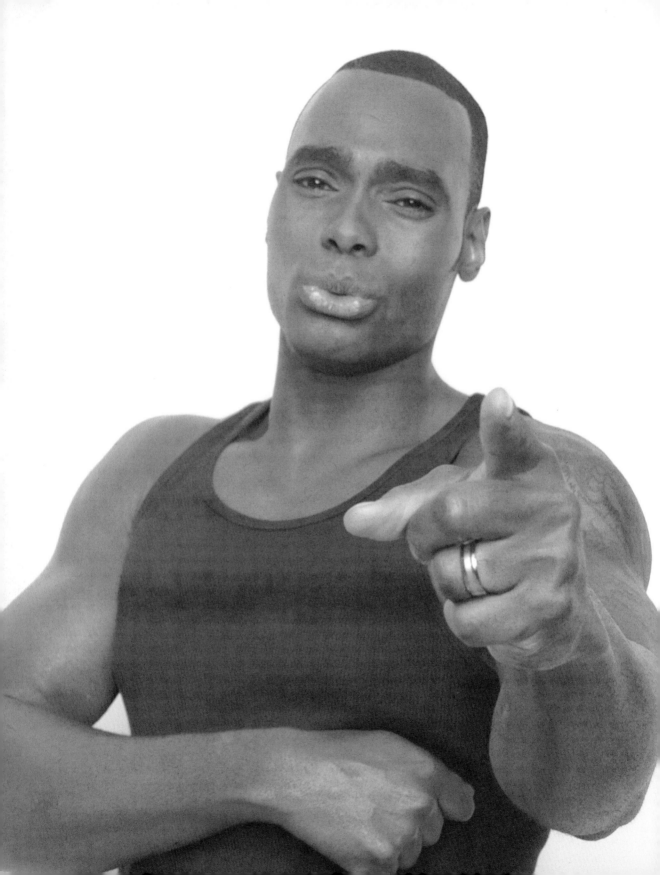

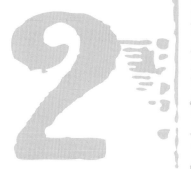

The Jump Off Philosophy

The first question you have to ask yourself is, Why am I reading this book? The second question is, Is that reason compelling enough for me to execute what's in the book? Perhaps you want a smaller waistline, or bigger arms, or tighter legs, but is that enough to sustain you through a 60-day transformation—and the rest of your life? Listen, I really want you to get something out of this, so I want you to go hard in your total transformation, maintain it, and perhaps inspire someone else.

No one exemplifies this hard-core approach better than Mary J. Blige. By the time I met her, she had already fired two trainers. She was resistant to me too at first, but I earned her respect and trust by doing what I promised to do, and I produced results to back it up. Once we got going, she was for real when it came to discipline. I find that this is a common denominator with all of the successful people that I train. Along with her talent, that's what made Mary a multiplatinum artist: d-i-s-c-i-p-l-i-n-e. Here's a woman who defines the word *diva,* but when it comes time to train, she'll push herself as hard as any male client would. She's not trying to look cute in the gym, either; it's all about the workout. She takes a chef with her now on tour just so she can focus on the diet! She bought into the fitness lifestyle to look better, but also to better herself personally and professionally.

Like Mary, you need to find a deeper reason to do this than just looking good—something that will hold you down when you feel like quitting. I've seen clients' whole lives change once they got their health and appearance issues right. Their increased confidence, improved energy, and hunger for living was incredible to see, and really beautiful to experience. I felt it and I want you to feel it. No matter what shape you are in, you can make improvements. Everyone can. This is your time. You can change your story.

As you get in shape, you'll find your quality of life improving. You'll be less fatigued. You'll be able to push that much harder, and look good while you're doing it. You'll also find that you have more intensity and more drive in your life. You'll have more internal control, and that will give you more control over the situations you encounter in your everyday life.

These changes will affect not only you but also those around you. You'll be more effective at providing for your loved ones because you'll have more energy and more focus. You'll be able to live longer and healthier, giving you more time to pursue your dreams. By starting this program, you're giving yourself the chance to live life to the fullest.

Your Story

We all have a story, and while everyone's story is different, they are also the same. What I mean by that is we all have a need for love and acceptance, and we all struggle with fears and insecurities.

I specialize in helping people in their struggles with health and hang-ups about their bodies. The first thing I tell each of my clients is that, with the right approach, you can improve your body and your health, no matter what shape you're in when you start. Often, people like to believe that circumstances are beyond their control. Why? Because when you believe that you don't have the power to change, then there's nothing you can do about your situation—and you don't have to take responsibility for changing it.

It's an easy out, and we've all done it. But there *is* an alternative. My job is to convince you that you do have control and you can change your life. Not to BS you, but to inspire you with some real talk and back that up with proof. Just look at my clientele. In 60 days, you can transform your physique—and your life.

Understand your story, but don't let it trap you. Know that it's only your current situation. For example, I have had clients say to me, right before a session, "I look like hell. I'm fat, Mark. I'm out of shape. What do I do?" They're sabotaging themselves at the very time they should be patting themselves on the back for making it to the session. The key to changing yourself is redefining your story. Instead of saying that you're fat, that you look like hell, that you have no will power, how about this? "I know I fell off last week, but today I'm totally focused, and I'm on it." Make this your story: "I'm losing weight; I look better than I did a couple of weeks ago. Sometimes I have trouble controlling my appetite, but, in knowing that, I can put more attention on that part of my life, and strive for improvement." Positive reinforcement is key.

It sounds simple. It is simple. You begin to change your story by *deciding* to change your story. So in starting this program, think about what your old story is, but think of it as a place you're leaving behind. Your new story is the journey that's going to take you where you want to go. Just by reading this book, you are taking the right steps.

The Jump Off program allows you to create this new story. It's a 60-day program, but you should see results within two weeks. By day 30, you should look pretty good. By day 60, you should be fresh! If you want this, show me something. Give me your all, and you'll be amazed at how quickly you get there.

My Story

Here's how I did it.

I was a fat kid. Back then I thought, "I am fat. My parents gave me bad eating habits. My mom didn't expose me to sports. I'm a middle child. My stepdad hates me. My mom doesn't care. Metabolism is bad. I don't have the time it would take to improve myself." Wah, wah, wah. I had a pity party every day, ending with dessert. As a result, I developed a lot of terrible eating habits. Then, in the military, I discovered that victory in every endeavor lies in honesty and perseverance. As long as you're still striving, you're still in the game, so keep at it.

Today, my story is far different than it used to be. Now I try to inspire others to be accountable for their health and their lives. I'm healthy and fit, but more importantly, so are those around me. My mother, my wife, and my in-laws are all much more health-conscious because of the example I set. Nothing makes me happier than knowing that those I love are healthy and taking control, and they're doing what it takes to live long, healthy, productive lives. This is the real reason for working out and committing to the fitness lifestyle. Pow!

Commitment and Motivation

Getting started is about wanting the 100 percent *you*, leaving no room for excuses. If you're tired of settling for less than 100 percent, then walk with me. Change your life! Forget about the past and the future, and think about *right now*.

In a sense, you're your own trainer. I may train clients, but they're the ones who make it happen. I consider myself to be one of the best, but all I can do is show up and tell them what to do. For this to work, we need to be a team. If you commit and promise to work with me, like Mary did, you'll see that there are no such things as obstacles—only opportunities to better yourself.

Do what it takes, and don't let your minor setbacks throw you off track. If you eat a piece of cake or miss a session, don't think: *Now I've messed up on my diet, so I'm going to cheat all day.* Or, *I've ducked a training session, so I'm not going to train all week.* Thinking that way only gives you permission to fall back into negative habits. Instead, use these slipups for motivation by making them part of your commitment. Everyone has setbacks, so don't get bogged down. Forgive yourself and use it as a way to deepen your commitment: *I ate some*

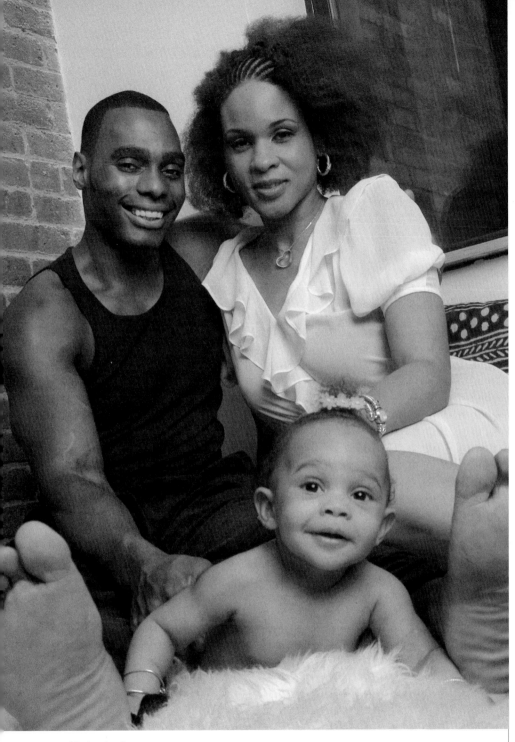

My inspirations.

cake yesterday, and it was good, but for the rest of the week, my diet is going to be flawless. Or, *I skipped the gym yesterday, but today I'm going to make up for it by training like an animal.* Say it and mean it. That's how you train yourself to win. It starts with a thought, then you verbalize it, and then you do it. Thought, word, deed.

Use that knowledge to your advantage and your results are guaranteed. You'll only need three to four hours a week, so, please, don't give me that I-don't-have-time story. How much TV do you watch each week? *Make* the time. Find out why celebs and CEOs are finding time to live the health-and-fitness lifestyle. Find out why they make time in their hectic schedules to ensure their health and longevity. Just look at Diddy—he ran a marathon. Johnnie Cochran's schedule is the most demanding I've seen, and he still finds time to fit in that workout by doing it at five o'clock in the morning.

Your Workout Program

Workout programs are as individual as you are, and I'm here to teach you how to take any workout program and customize it to fit your individual needs. In doing so, you need to balance two things.

1. What you need to do (exercises you usually don't like doing)
2. What you want to do (exercises you like doing)

If you set up a program that you hate, even if it's exactly what you need, you're setting yourself up for failure. You might do it for 30 days, or even 60, but if you're miserable, you'll run out of steam soon enough. If every exercise targets something you're weak at, you'll never stay the course. You have to do some exercises you like so that you stay psyched up and into the workout. You need that feeling of accomplishment after every workout.

At the same time, don't do only what you love to do. The exercises you're weak at will actually balance your body and produce the best results. That means Chest Masters, please work your legs, and Ab Masters, don't neglect your lower back. Maybe you like to do cardio on a rowing machine. Cool—include that. Maybe you hate to squat, even though you have thin legs.

Well, include squats, but don't feel like you have to do them every time you go to the gym, or even every time you train legs. Just make sure you hit them twice a month.

No one is going to be motivated every time they hit the gym if they're following a boring, corny routine. But you've got to do some of the dirty work to balance out that hard body! Everyone has body parts they hate to train, but each body part is important for total fitness, so leave no part untrained.

Every workout program should include these components: cardiovascular training, weight training (both lower and upper body, people!), and flexibility work. People who train on their own, without guidance, tend to eliminate one or more of these components, which is a huge mistake. Do it right! Train by the book.

Cardiovascular Training

No wonder the obesity rate in the United States climbs higher and higher. Everything is automated—cars, elevators, escalators, you name it. We overeat at work and then come home, sit down, and watch TV.

That's why cardio is huge. Not only does it burn calories, but it also improves the functioning of your body. It improves your heart as well as the efficiency of your lungs. It helps reduce cholesterol, burn body fat, control blood pressure, and build endurance.

Any sensible workout program absolutely needs to include cardio, but be careful not to OD. Some people want to do cardio and nothing else. Although they are lean, they have no muscle mass and are flabby. Slim-Flabs—that's what I call them. Their muscles have no tone because they don't include any resistance training in their program. They should not depend on any one aspect of training to control their weight, and neither should you. To win long-term, combine resistance training, cardio, and diet.

Be proactive about doing cardio, whether that means going for a brisk walk, using cardio equipment at the gym, going for a run or jog, playing tag with the kids, or using some of the more specific techniques I describe in the chapter devoted to cardiovascular training. Bottom line, you have to make time for this. We all need a healthy heart.

Resistance Training

A lot of people don't want to weight-train for a variety of reasons. Some avoid it because they think cardio is the be-all and end-all of weight loss. I just shot that myth down. A lot of my female clients are scared that weights will make them big and bulky, but this is just a misconception spread by people who lifted weights without dieting. Everyone needs resistance training, from children to senior citizens. Let me explain why.

The more muscular you are, the more calories you burn at rest. Every pound of muscle takes 10 calories to sustain. Muscle drives up your metabolic rate, allowing you to process calories more efficiently without storing them as body fat. You'll burn much more body fat if you perform cardio *and* weight-train than if you just do cardio alone.

When you weight-train, you will add a few pounds of muscle mass, but you'll also lose body fat. If you gain 10 pounds of muscle and only lose 8 pounds of fat, you'll look trimmer, even though technically you're 2 pounds heavier. You'll look tighter and stronger. Your waist size will diminish and your shoulders and back will be more tapered. In other words, it's not about how much you weigh, but how much body fat you're carrying around. You're better off evaluating yourself by how you look and feel than by reading numbers on a scale.

This goes for men and women. Women worry about getting muscular, but I'm here to tell you that it doesn't go down that way. They don't develop outrageously huge muscles from working out with dumbbells. What they do is get toned, taut, and sexy muscles. They get sculpted.

A couple of years ago, I had this client, a famous publicist, who didn't want to weight-train because she thought she looked like a brick instead of an hourglass. That was her old story, and she needed to trust the weights and her trainer to help chisel her new body. I designed a program focusing on narrowing her waist with diet and cardio, but building her shoulders, chest, and back with resistance training. By making her upper body a little more muscular and accentuating certain muscles, she was able to create the appearance of a much narrower waist and a curvier physique. When she saw her body changing, she was no longer controlled by her old body image. That's what weights can do for you. Pay attention—these are tricks of the trade.

Stretching

Flexibility is one of the most overlooked aspects of the average workout program. Nothing keeps your muscles, bones, and joints in better shape than regular stretching. Yet few workout books incorporate it, and very few people at the average gym stretch regularly. That sends the message that stretching isn't very important, but you're more likely to get injured if flexibility isn't part of your program. This is critical. A pulled muscle can sideline you for months.

Today, people have all sorts of overuse injuries from working at computers and performing other repetitive tasks. By keeping your body flexible, you can avoid many of these problems. When you're flexible, you move better, your posture is better, and your circulation is better. For the extratense businessman, the first thing I tell him is to go take a yoga class. This is one of the things I emphasized to P. Diddy. Because of the stressful nature of his work, he needs to focus on flexibility as much as on cardio and weight training.

When you stretch, you should always warm up first. Often, people think that stretching *is* warming up, but they're two different things. First, get your body temperature up on a treadmill or stationary bike (or go for a jog) for 5 to 10 minutes. Now when you stretch, your muscles will be much more flexible because they're warm and you'll be ready to attack the workout. They'll open up better, and you'll really reduce the chance of injuring yourself. You don't have to be superflexible, but you want to be flexible enough that you won't pull a muscle during the rest of your workout. You don't need to stretch for long: 5 to 10 minutes will suffice, going slightly beyond the range of motion you'll use in your workout.

The real stretching comes at the end of your workout, though. Stretch every muscle in your body, spending a little extra time stretching the muscles you just trained. This will help work out the lactic acid, reducing the amount of soreness you'll feel the next day and the extrastiff muscle-man look. Stretching is the key to having a safe workout and to helping the body recover from the rigors of training. Do not overlook this aspect or you'll pay for it later.

Getting With the Program

Although this book contains a detailed program for you to follow, never hesitate to include some variety. One mistake people make is relying too much on one type of training, perhaps even repeating the same workout endlessly. You may feel like you're making strides because you can press the same weight overhead for a rep or two more, but really your body is just getting used to the workload. It may feel like you're improving because you don't get sore, but that also means that you're not working your body as hard.

The body is quick to adapt, so always keep it off balance. The key is change. Don't hesitate to throw a new exercise into the mix. If it starts to get stale for you, change the order of your exercises from one workout to the next. Use heavier weights for fewer reps in one workout, then the next time drop the weight and perform as many reps as you can. All of these strategies will force your body to work harder. Keep your body guessing, and the results will keep coming. Vary your workouts, and your body will always respond.

Intensity

If you aren't training hard, or if you're just going through the motions, you're not getting the most out of your time. When I train clients, I help them crank up the intensity as high as possible. Other than Mary J. Blige and Diddy, who are both animals, almost every celebrity client of mine has thrown up at one time or another. I train them this hard so that when our time is up and they start training by themselves, they'll know what 100 percent feels like.

Keep it real with yourself about how hard you're pushing it. When I taught in New York, I had the most popular jump-rope class because of the intensity. I even brought in African drummers so the class wasn't limited by the speed of the music. If you wanted to step it up, then the drummers automatically started beating faster. This is what you have to do when you're training yourself. Ask yourself, Did I use as much weight as I could have? Did I run as far as I could have? Make sure you go all out, and you can't lose. The object isn't to finish the class. It is to survive for as long as you can, and then go a minute longer than that the next class.

It's up to you to find what drives your intensity. Maybe it's music. Maybe it's positive reinforcement. Maybe it's rewarding yourself (although not in a way that undermines your hard work). Maybe it's negative reinforcement: "If I don't lift this weight with perfect form for 10 reps, then I'm going to do an extra 20 minutes on the treadmill." Maybe it's visualization or taking pictures of your body every two weeks. Find out what it takes to motivate yourself with the intensity that you need to succeed. I know you can do it, but no one knows what drives you better than you.

Your Nutrition Program

The funny thing about nutrition is that, like your story, everybody is different and everybody is the same. Certain rules apply to some individuals, and some rules apply to everyone. But body types fall into one of three general categories:

* ✳ *Endomorphs:* People who tend to hold a lot of fat. (Me. My body type. Damn!) Another celebrity example is D'Angelo.
* ✳ *Mesomorphs:* People who tend to be lean and have muscles. You know those folks who look good without ever touching a weight? They're mesos. (They drive me crazy, and I want to discuss them no further.) LL exemplifies this body type.
* ✳ *Ectomorphs:* People who tend to be skinny—naturally lean with little muscle. You know, the ones who can eat anything and still look skinny. (I hate them, too.) Chris Rock and Kelly Rowland of Destiny's Child are examples of this look.

Endomorphs have to watch their food consumption more carefully than the other types. At the other extreme, ectomorphs may need to consume more than they naturally want to eat just to keep their weight up. This is especially true when you burn more calories by exercising.

The Basics

Food consists of three basic nutrients: fat, carbohydrate, and protein. How much of each you should eat depends on several factors, but keep in mind that calories count. The unit of measurement for energy or heat is the calorie: (1 calorie represents the amount of heat needed to raise the temperature of 1 gram of water 1 degree Celsius. Only macronutrients—as opposed to water, fiber, vitamins, and minerals—contain calories. Carbohydrate and protein both have 4 calories per gram, fat has 9, and alcohol has 7. If you're trying to lose body fat, you need to eat fewer calories than it takes for your body to maintain its weight. If you want to add muscle mass, more likely you'll need to eat more than it takes for maintenance (unless you're also trying to lose body fat at the same time).

Here are some basics. For more detail on my nutrition program, turn to Chapter 7.

Protein. To build muscle mass, you need to provide your body with amino acids, the building blocks of protein. When you consume protein, your body breaks it back down into aminos to build and repair muscle mass. When you don't eat protein, your body tears down existing muscle mass to acquire the aminos necessary to repair the muscle tissue. Basically, you're feeding off your own muscle. This is counterproductive. Consuming plenty of protein is the answer.

This protein should be equally divided over five or six meals. That's right: five or six meals a day. But hold on—more about that in a minute.

Carbohydrate. This nutrient is the trickiest element of any diet to manage, which is one reason it's in all the headlines. Consume too few and you'll feel brain-dead. Consume too many and you won't be able to see your feet in the shower.

Carbohydrate consumption should be front-loaded, meaning feast on them in the morning, especially during breakfast, and then taper off as your day unfolds. Just to give you an example, I eat as much as 75 percent of my carb calories with breakfast. (I eat the rest after my workout.) After essentially fasting overnight, your body craves energy food. Carbs such as those found in oatmeal or pancakes—whole wheat, that is—can be converted into slow-burning energy that will keep you energized for hours with minimal fat storage.

In Chapter 7, I'll give you detailed information on these and other carb sources. You'll learn which ones to avoid, as well as how to incorporate good carbs into your diet.

Fat. Dietary fat doesn't make you fat—excess calories do. As long as you're keeping your calories in check, you can eat dietary fat. In fact, many fat-containing foods are extremely healthy. Salmon, olives, avocados, nuts and seeds, and oils such as olive, canola, and flax seed all contain healthy fats. These can actually help you lose body fat and lower cholesterol.

What you want to avoid are saturated and trans fats, which are found in fried foods, desserts, margarine, butter, mayonnaise, and fatty red meats. These are high in calories and will clog your arteries. Straight up, these are among the worst foods out there. Many of them should come with a Surgeon General's warning, because they will kill you over time. Don't think you have to avoid meat altogether, though. Au contraire: many sources are lean and mean, such as chicken breast, turkey breast, ostrich, buffalo, white fish, and the best cuts of beef. While they contain some saturated fats, they're a good source of protein, especially when you consider the low number of calories they contain.

Meal Magic

One of the most important elements of a healthy nutrition program is eating many meals a day. At first it may sound crazy, but you're much more likely to lose body fat if you eat more often.

In fact, I recommend eating five or six times a day. Here's why: each regular-sized meal takes about 100 calories simply to digest. If you split the same amount of food you're eating over five or six meals as you would normally eat in three, then you're burning 600 versus 300 calories a day just digesting your food. That alone gives you a calorie deficit of 300—almost an hour on the treadmill. Imagine getting ripped by eating more frequently!

Frequent meals also provide your body with a constant source of the protein necessary for building muscle, provided you eat protein at each meal. They also provide a steady stream of energy (from carbs and fat) that keep your blood sugar steady, so your body will stay energized and continue metabolizing body fat.

Of course, eating five meals a day can be an overwhelming amount of food to prepare—and expensive—so I suggest drinking two to three protein shakes a day on top of three small food meals. If you want to get in shape quickly, shakes can be your best friend. Not only can they give you the protein you need, but they also allow you to control calories. This makes the numbers a lot easier to hit when you're trying to keep calories down and protein up and you don't have the time to cook. Be careful when you're hitting those shakes to make sure that your protein powder has enough fiber, though. Again, you can't beat the bang for the buck.

Water

Then there's water, one of the most overlooked elements of a healthy lifestyle. I can't overstate the importance of drinking this liquid gold. If you don't drink enough, you aren't as healthy as you could be, and your body isn't functioning at maximum capacity. Water also helps flush out toxins and waste material that will otherwise stay inside you, looking for an opportunity to cause trouble.

Water also gives muscle cells what they need to do their thing: grow. It's crucial for helping your body process protein. A protein-packed diet is not harmful to a healthy person, but this muscle-building macronutrient is easily processed if you drink enough water.

Everyone reading this book should be drinking a *minimum* of eight 8-ounce glasses of water a day. When you work out, you sweat, and when you sweat, you need even more fluids. So you should also drink about 16 ounces of water in the half hour or so before a workout. Drink plenty of water during the workout, too.

Keep in mind that certain drinks, like caffeinated coffee, and particularly alcohol, are very dehydrating. When you consume these liquids, increase water consumption above the baseline recommended here. All in all, I recommend that active people take in a gallon of water a day. You may go to the bathroom more, but you'll live longer. Not a bad deal, huh?

Cheating

It's not realistic to think that once you start this program, you're never going to cheat. Even I fall off the wagon once in a while. I'm a former fat kid, so when I cheat, it gets ugly.

When it comes to staying on your diet, everybody has good and bad days. The key is to know your limits, and to factor at least some backsliding into your program, especially during the holidays. The worst thing you can do is to start having self-sabotaging thoughts when you cheat. Just because you had a banana split, don't think, *Man, I blew it. I ruined my program. There's no point in continuing.* If you think that way, you'll never change your story and become the new you. Refocus. Instead, think, *That pie was good, but now I'm going to have to be really dedicated to reach my goals. I'll eat properly today and the next day.* Then, commit to it meal by meal. Get back on it. Reconfirm your personal goal.

Including a small element of cheating in your diet right out of the gate can keep backsliding from becoming failure. Over the weekend, factor in a piece of pie. Eat a few slices of pizza (just use a napkin to absorb some of the excess grease beforehand). When you know you're going to eat a big dinner, reduce your carbs throughout the day so that you don't have a whole bunch of carbs in your stomach when you hit the sack. Stay focused and be reasonable. Schedule your cheating before you get critical. Don't wait till you're in savage beast mode to start looking for garbage to eat.

Food and Emotion

In order to stay on course, learn to detach yourself from food. In my opinion, food is the biggest drug on the streets. When people feel bad, they eat food to cheer themselves up. When people feel good, they eat food to celebrate. When people are bored, they eat just to be eatin'.

Remember, food is meant for nourishment. Consumed wisely, it allows you to derive the most pleasure possible from all other areas of your life. It should be a means of getting you to your goal, not the goal itself. Don't get me wrong, because I love to eat just as much as the next guy. It's all about putting food in perspective. A couple of weeks of indulgence can take months or even years to work off. In the long run, it ain't worth it.

To stay in shape for the long haul, look at food as fuel and yourself as a finely tuned set of wheels. You wouldn't put just any junk in the tank of a Ferrari, would you? And even if you did, that beautiful ride would choke along like a hooptie. I find it interesting that most people treat their bodies worse than their cars. You make sure it's gassed, you make sure the fluids are right, you make sure the chassis is clean—why don't you do the same for your body? It's not that difficult to get in shape, but being in shape for a lifetime requires as much mental concentration as it does physical effort.

I often have my clients write down their emotions as well as the foods they're eating so that they can see the relationship right in front of them in black and white. Oftentimes, the worst eating habits go along with negative emotions such as depression, fear, anger, and frustration. Sometimes people overeat to mask their real problems—I know I used to. Analyze yourself, your habits, and your motives. Be honest with yourself, and then take action, whether it's therapy, exercise, or a combination of both.

The Fat-Loss Control Mechanism

Cardio is great for helping you get in shape, but I don't like to see my clients use it as their primary means of controlling weight. You shouldn't have the mind-set that you're going to go do 90 minutes of cardio to burn calories just to stay even. This sets you up for disaster. First, it's compulsive. Second, it's unsustainable. Eventually, you will fall off your daily half-marathon, and the weight will catch up with you. Another disadvantage is that doing too much cardio can burn up precious muscle mass. When you go wild with cardio, you train your body to preferentially burn muscle mass over body fat. Essentially, you retard your metabolism.

Before I trained Missy Elliott, she went on the treadmill after every meal. Considering the impact that constant pounding was having on her joints, no wonder why her knees hurt all the time.

So it's always better to use your diet rather than your cardio to control your body weight. You're always in control of how much food you put into your body. On days when you know that your caloric expenditure is not going to be as high as others, cut back on the amount of food you take in. By using common sense and paying attention to your body and your emotional state, you can really make the Jump Off work for you.

Tying It All Together

In addition to diet and training, other elements can help keep you focused and working toward your goal. In fact, I highly recommend doing all of the following:

> *1. Keep journals. In addition to writing down all your exercise (sets, reps, exercises performed, and your cardio with times and intensity) and your*

nutrition (all your foods at every meal, including snacks), you should also record all the emotions and events relevant to your program.

If you're having a bad day, record your mind-set, whether you're feeling angry, frustrated, depressed, or some other emotion entirely. Try to articulate why you feel that way. Do the same on good days. This helps you to understand yourself, and the better you understand the man or woman in the mirror, the better you'll function as your own trainer and motivator.

When you see that on Tuesday you ate three pieces of cake, and recorded that you were depressed, you'll start to identify your self-sabotaging behaviors. You'll start to recognize that when you feel a particular emotion, you really have to be cautious and stave off the negative behaviors that usually accompany it.

That's not to say you won't feel unhappy or depressed sometimes. We all do. What you're trying to do is identify these occurrences before you fall off the wagon and wreck your program. Recognize that you feel badly, and then do what you can to control the damage. You'll be that much more ahead of the game, and you'll avoid situations that could derail your progress.

Having your journal is the key to understanding yourself and developing that self-control that comes with self-realization.

2. Breathe properly. Just as many people don't drink enough water, many people don't breathe properly. Water and air are the two things we need most for survival, and yet we take them for granted.

Breathing deeply is important for health. It improves your lung capacity, reduces your heart rate, and helps you relax. Try this experiment: Take five long, slow breaths right now, pulling as much air as you can into your lungs. Hold each breath, then expel it. Feel more relaxed? That's what you're missing if you're not breathing deeply.

Many go through life without ever doing this. Life is often stressful, and people constantly react by taking shallow breaths and then puffing them out. Ironically, smokers often breathe in deeply when they inhale their cigarettes. That's all part of the reinforcement of the addiction.

Breathing deeply feels good, and smokers often transfer that feeling to the cigarettes.

When you perform your exercises, think about your breathing and use it to control your focus and your heart rate. This has a very purifying effect on the body, mind, and spirit. Remember, deep breathing plus water equals healthy mind and body.

3. Don't neglect your spirituality. *Finally, incorporate an element of the spiritual into your program. This will mean something different to each person, but it will have a similar cleansing effect on everyone. Decide what the spiritual aspect of your program is, whether it's meditation, a morning ritual, a massage, a soak in a hot bath, or your acknowledgement of a higher power. Rededicate yourself to this spiritual element every day. When you pay attention to your spiritual needs, you take care of the vessel that houses your soul. Spiritual development will keep you on the path, even when you falter physically and mentally.*

Also, spirituality helps to keep you humble. I know you know someone who's in great shape, yet acts like a jerk because he or she is in great shape. This attitude turns off a lot of people to the fitness lifestyle. These people focus too much on the external without putting energy into the spiritual element. It's all about finding that balance.

I know that's a lot to digest while you're sitting here reading. As you read certain passages, you might be thinking, *What the heck is he talking about? I thought this was a hip-hop hard-body manual.* This is a good thing. I want you to explore and find out the truth for yourself. A large portion of this book won't make sense until you start your quest to release the real you that's deep down inside. You'll see that all the information here is essential. I wanted to give you the same lessons I give to all of my clients. Your program is not about getting your body right. It's about the changes that happen during the process of getting your body right. It's not about your goal; it's about your journey.

Get Started

Assuming you've worked out before, remember the first time you felt like you were really making some progress? Maybe it was the day you racked those 5-pound dumbbells and opted for 10s instead. Perhaps it was when you felt a real pump for the first time. Or maybe it was the day you caught a sidelong glance from the handsome guy or cute girl on the next bench—you know, the one who wouldn't give you the time of day three months prior. Those were all tantalizing clues that your body was beginning to undergo some sort of transformation.

Felt pretty good, didn't it?

If you've been there before, I'm going to help you recapture that feeling. If you haven't felt it before, you're about to feel it for the first time. You have my personal guarantee on that. In either case, experiencing that feeling isn't the destination. It's the starting line for a lifelong race toward something much greater: your personal best.

The workouts we're going to use to accomplish that are probably unlike anything you've seen or done before. If you're looking for the same ol', same ol', you've come to the wrong place. What you will find here are three workouts that are highly efficient, highly effective, challenging, and, most of all, fun.

But I have to warn you, these workouts are not easy. Nothing worth doing is. The upper-body, lower-body, flexibility, and outdoor workouts are based on university studies and 10 years of my own experience with training clients. These are the same workouts I use on celebs.

Not only is variety the spice of life, it's also the key to a good workout program. If you equate working out with doing 20 sets of bench presses or two hours of cardio, you're in for a shock. In typical weight training, you use what's called your anaerobic energy system, which fuels short bursts of strength. In typical cardio, you're using your aerobic system, which relies on oxygen for a more sustained effort.

Here, you'll be switching back and forth between the two in a new, unique way. In between conventional resistance-training exercises like the dumbbell overhead press, you'll be doing activities like jumping jacks and boxing drills. The drills are strategically placed in the middle of the lifting to keep your heart rate elevated and moving from start to finish. I want you to burn fat, build muscle, and pump it up at the same time. The workouts in *The Jump Off* will get you to the killer hard-body in record time!

Use the element of surprise on your own body. Where training is concerned, shock is good. Your body builds muscle in response to fibers being hit with new and different stimuli. The trick is that your body only changes when it's forced to, and it's remarkably quick to adapt. If you repeat the same workout every training session even for three months, your body will adapt and your gains will slow. If you feel like your progress has reached a plateau, this is probably what's happening.

So keep your body guessing, and don't be afraid to put on a little muscle, which is the best thing you can do to burn fat. Muscle is the most metabolically active tissue in the human body, meaning it burns the most calories internally. The more muscle you have, the more efficient your body becomes at burning fat, even when you're sleeping! When I put LL through his paces, he never knew what to expect. One leg day, squats; the next leg day, uphill sprints. Did it work? You've seen him. You tell me.

Quality is better than quantity. Many beginners overdo it under the assumption that more is better, especially when results first appear. However, you're much better off focusing on three to four hard-core sessions per week than on hitting the gym every day, which will burn you out sooner or later. Challenge yourself each workout, instead of working out constantly. You want to feel psyched about your next workout, not annoyed that you have to go. Go hard, diet, and rest.

Recovery is just as important as training. When you lift weights, you're actually tearing down muscle fibers. It's only after you've completed your workout that your muscle tissues begin rebuilding. For that to go down smoothly, it's critical to have downtime between workouts. Beginners in particular shouldn't lift more than three or four times a week. Nor should they work the same muscle group on consecutive days. Most importantly, they should never train a muscle group that's still sore from a prior workout.

A great workout doesn't require a bunch of crazy or expensive equipment. All you really need to do these workouts is a set of dumbbells and an exercise ball. I've designed them so that you can do them at home as easily as you can in the gym. And let's face it: After a tough day at work, maybe followed by a few hours of parenting, getting in the car and heading off to the gym isn't always a desirable or realistic scenario.

(By the way, I get all of my exercise equipment—parachutes, stability balls, and dumbbells—from performbetter.com. They'll get it to you quickly and it's cheap.)

Don't get discouraged as your rate of progress slows. When you first start training, results can come quickly. That pace will diminish, but don't let that throw you for a loop. It's like anything in life: the better you get, the harder it is to improve. So use this as motivation to work out and diet harder, rather than getting discouraged. It just goes to show you that the human body can adapt to almost anything, and as it adapts, further progress becomes that much harder to generate. What that boils down to is, the better shape you're in, the harder you have to train to make it happen. But don't get discouraged; just keep attacking.

Adjust as necessary. Don't do your sets mindlessly. Keep an eye on the progress you're making, particularly as it's reflected in your body. Look at your symmetry. If your chest is lagging behind other parts of your body, by all means, do an extra 15 reps for your chest. Focus on the areas that you want to prioritize. Sculpt that body!

Your life involves a lot more than just getting to the gym, so plan accordingly. Your workouts need to be efficient—no, superefficient. I don't want you in the gym a minute longer than necessary, and I don't want to waste it by making you do a single unneeded repetition. I really want you to get in, push the workout, and get out. *The Jump Off* asks you to work out three times a week, with each workout lasting 45 minutes to an hour. Based on my experience, most people with jobs and families don't have the mental focus, physical stamina, or recovery ability to train effectively for longer than that. Most people who claim to spend two or three hours in the gym spend half that time socializing. You're not there to make friends. At least, wait till after your workout to start rapping.

A full-body workout might be a good training introduction for a complete new-comer, or for someone who's insanely busy, but the best results come when you divide your workout into training specific parts. It's called a training split, and that's what you're going to be doing here. Because you won't be training your entire body on the same day, you can devote more focused attention to the part or parts that you *are* training. It's also a good way to give your body more time to recover and grow. Therein lies the beauty of a split system: the parts of your body that you just worked get plenty of R&R as the days unfold and you move on to your other body parts. In fact, it's best if your training days aren't consecutive. Placing 24 hours between sessions is a great idea.

A training split can assume many forms, but after years of experimentation, I've come up with a unique approach as simple as it is effective. I devote one day to upper body, another day to lower body, and a third day to outdoor training that works the full body along with improving cardiovascular endurance.

Sound cool? Then what are you waiting for? Turn the page, start your mission, and release the beast!

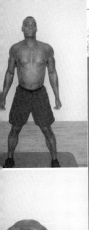

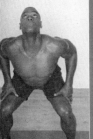

THE JUMP OFF PROGRAM 2

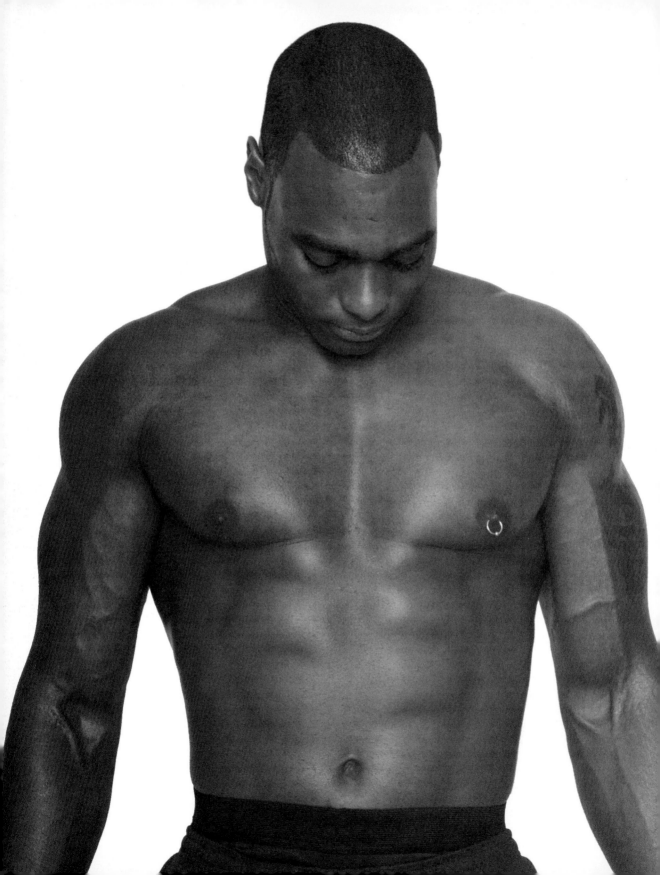

The Upper-Body Attack

I know you can't wait to get started, but before we delve into Day One, the upper-body attack, let me lay a few ground rules on you.

Rule 1: Always warm up your muscles before training them. This one simple step will improve your workouts and prevent injuries. A mere five minutes spent on a cardio machine using your large muscles, particularly your legs—even if that's not what you're training that day—is an adequate warm-up. That's why we start with the jump rope!

Rule 2: Stretch after warm-up and before, during, and after working out. This post-work-out training session, done when your muscles are warm and elastic, is a great way to promote maximum recovery and extend your range of motion. Stretches should be static (don't bounce) and held for a count of 10 to 15 seconds apiece.

Rule 3: Keep up the tempo. After finishing with chest or any other body part, rest just long enough for a quick stretch and a drink of water. Then move on immediately to the next body part. Be serious! Watch the clock. Try to get your workouts done within an hour, and then cut two minutes off successive sessions until you're down to 45 minutes or so.

Enough talk. Let's get busy? Here's today's workout.

The Upper-Body Workout

EXERCISE	SETS	REPS/TIME
Chest		
1. Jumping rope	1	100 skips or 5 minutes (This is designed to warm you up as much as it is to work these body parts.)
2. Push-up on ball	3	10–20 reps
3. Incline flye on ball	3	15–20 reps
Shoulders		
4. Overhead dumbbell press	3	15–30 reps
5. Weighted boxing jabs	1	100 jabs each arm, 20 at a time; or 3 minutes (1 round!)
Back		
6. Deadlift-row	3	10–20 reps
7. Reverse hyperextension	3	10–20 reps
8. Football footwork drill	100	Patter steps (Speed—we need speed!)

Arms

9. Dumbbell curl	3	15–30 reps
10. Dumbbell kickback	3	15–30 reps
11. Jumping jacks	1	100 (Old school exercise!)

Core

(Don't stop! You're almost done! Finish in less than an hour!)

12. Ball crunch	1	30–60 reps
13. Ball twist	1	30–60 reps
14. Ball tuck	1	30 reps

Chest

For some men and women, especially, training themselves can be intimidating, but you're going to soldier through. The intimidation factor is particularly high when you're training chest. Try to visualize the muscle contracting as you train. The more you put your mind to the muscle, the better your results will be. A strong chest is a must for posture and is pleasing to the eye as well. This applies to both sexes. For men, it gives you a powerful look; for women, it accentuates your curves. Think about the muscle and squeeze. Stay in control. No sloppy form!

1. JUMPING ROPE

WHY YOU'RE DOING IT: The main goals here are to get your heart rate elevated and to warm up your shoulder joints for the pressing movements to follow.

HOW TO DO IT: Everyone has probably jumped rope at some point in his or her life, but not everyone has done it correctly. The most important thing is to choose a rope that's long enough. Put your foot down on the middle of the rope, and then pull the ends up toward you. If the rope is long enough, the ends will reach up to your chest. Once you begin jumping, keep your elbows in toward your sides. Remember, you only have to jump as high as the rope is thick.

The drill:

Five minutes, or 100 skips. Five minutes equals 2 miles. Get to work, baby!

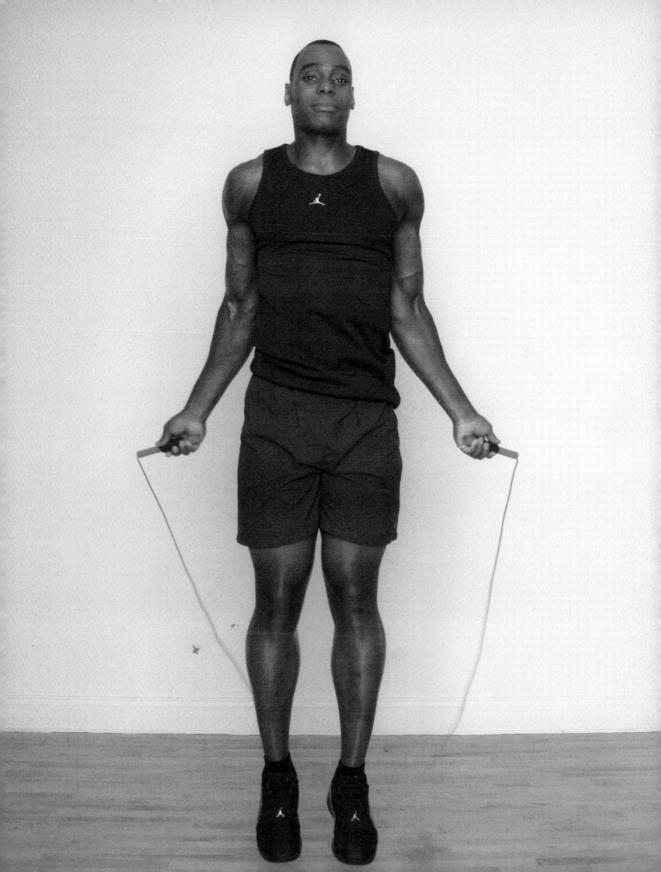

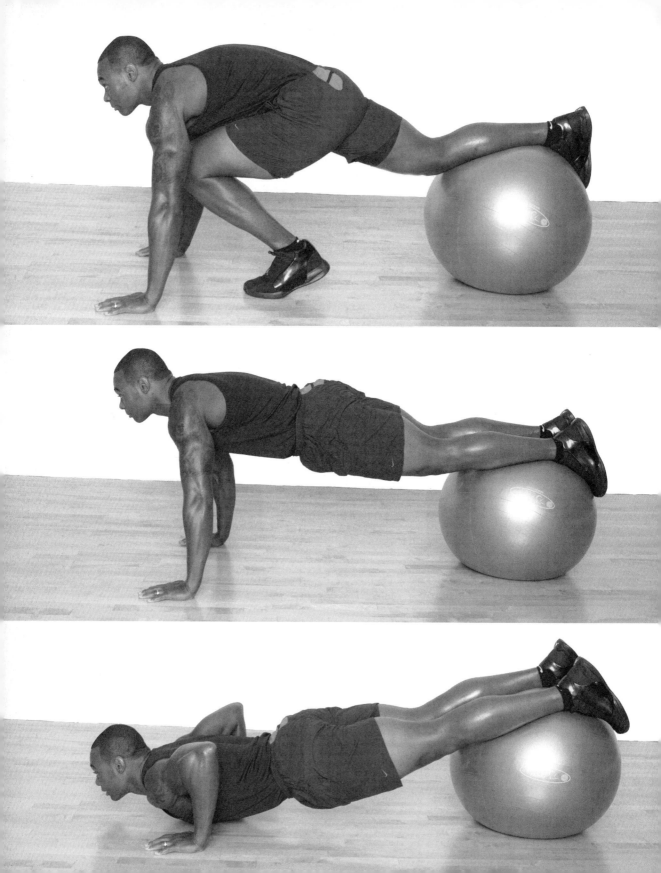

2. PUSH-UP ON BALL

WHY YOU'RE DOING IT: The push-up is a great exercise to begin with, but using the exercise ball makes it better still. Whereas the traditional push-up mimics the flat bench press, elevating your feet makes it more closely resemble the incline bench press. That means you're getting more involvement from the upper pecs and front delts.

The difficulty increases due to the different angle and the loss of stability on the ball, assuming you keep most of your lower legs off the ball. If you find this version hard at first, decrease the difficulty by having more of your legs supported by the ball. This decreases the length of the lever (that is, your total body length, or where the pivoting occurs). Or you can do the traditional push-up if this is too advanced for you. If that's still too hard, you can do push-ups off your knees. No excuses—make it happen!

HOW TO DO IT: Lie face down with your elbows bent; your hands a few inches from your sides, just below chest level, and your feet elevated on an exercise ball. Push your body off the floor, rising until your arms are extended (but don't lock your elbows). Bend your elbows to lower your torso back down to the starting position. Your head, back, and hips should stay aligned throughout the movement.

The drill:
Three sets, 10 to 20 reps. Go get it!

3. INCLINE FLYE ON BALL

WHY YOU'RE DOING IT: To look sexy and strong from the front—why else?

HOW TO DO IT: Lie face up across an exercise ball, holding a dumbbell in each hand, so that your chest is higher than your butt. Extend your arms straight overhead so that the dumbbells touch and your palms face each other. From this starting position, allow the dumbbells to travel out and downward in an arc. Keep your elbows slightly bent and locked as they descend so that at the bottom your palms are facing the ceiling and your wrists are flexed slightly. Bring the weights up in front of you in an arc until they come together, maintaining the constant bend in your elbows.

The drill:
Three sets, 15 to 20 reps. Embrace the pain. Exhale as you squeeze!

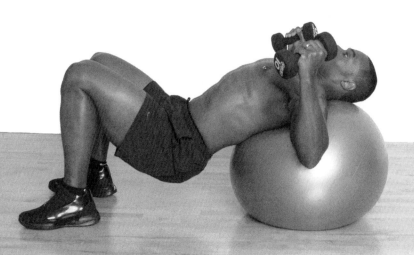

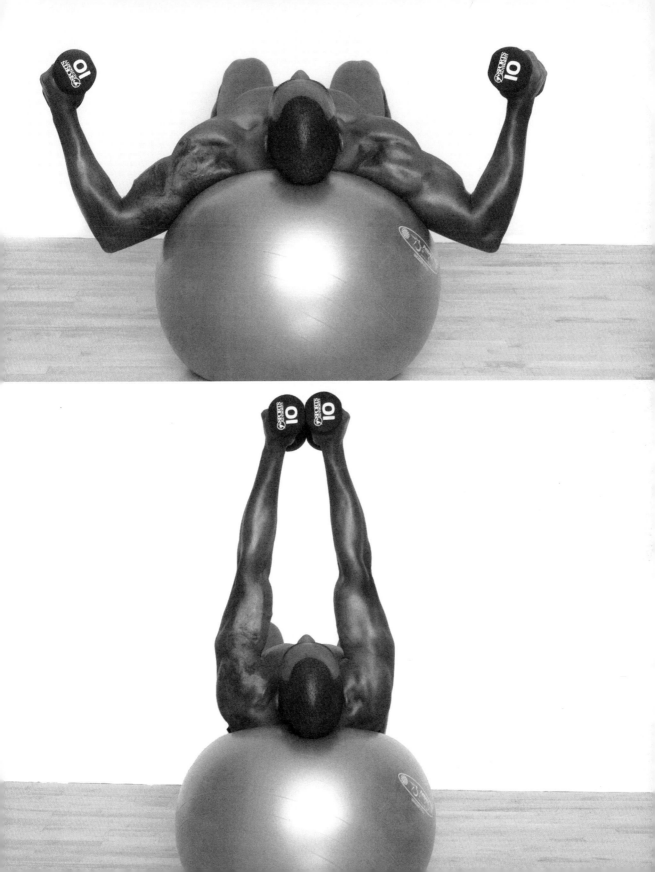

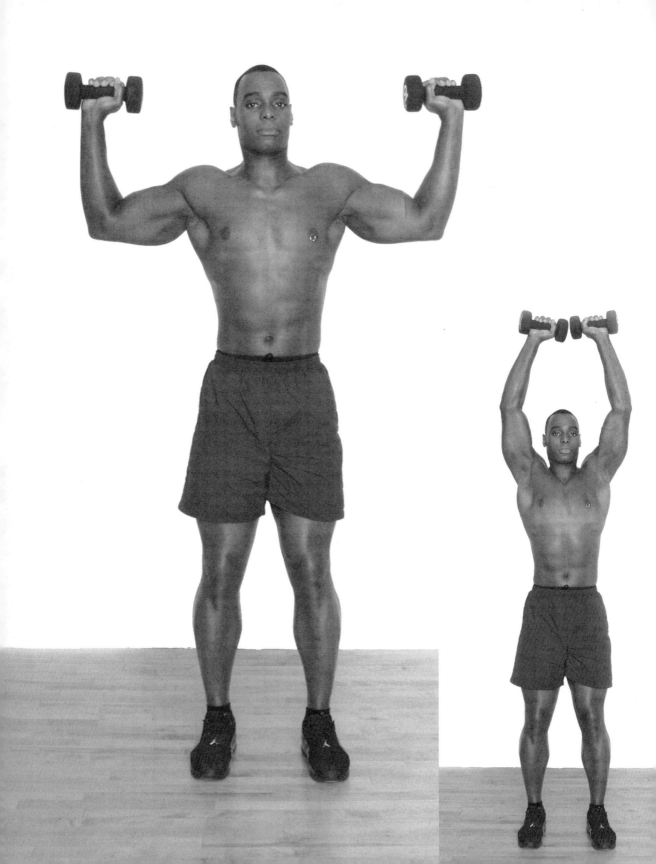

Shoulders

Clothes make the man (and woman), but shoulders make the clothes. Sure, abs receive more attention on the beach and at the newsstand, but aren't those the only places where you actually *see* a six-pack exposed? When it comes to your appearance, shoulders reign supreme. As soon as someone sees your body from head to toe, a judgment has been passed as to your shoulder-to-waist ratio.

The textbook term for the shoulder muscle is the *deltoid*, and each of yours has three separate heads: the front, the middle, and the rear. Because the shoulder complex consists of those three muscle heads, I made sure the Jump Off hits them all.

4. OVERHEAD DUMBBELL PRESS

WHY YOU'RE DOING IT: This is great for working the entire shoulder but especially the front and side heads. I prefer dumbbells to barbells for these because they allow you to use the range of motion that feels most comfortable, and they promote even arm development; one can't compensate for the other as with barbells.

HOW TO DO IT: Stand holding dumbbells in each hand. Assume the starting position by raising the dumbbells to shoulder level, in a goal-post formation, with your palms facing forward. Keeping your back straight and your feet planted firmly, press the dumbbells overhead simultaneously, more or less straight up. At the top, give your shoulder muscles a little squeeze, and slowly lower the dumbbells back to the starting position.

The drill:
Three sets, 15 to 30 reps.

5. WEIGHTED BOXING JABS

WHY YOU'RE DOING IT: To keep your heart rate elevated and to fry those shoulders.

HOW TO DO IT: Picture Muhammad Ali shadowboxing, and you'll have a good idea of how to perform these. Stay on the balls of your feet and extend your elbows to throw rapid-fire punches. Punch as you step. Keep your feet moving throughout. You can use dumbbells or not. Just work it. (Rocky theme music is optional.)

The drill:
100 jabs each arm, 20 at a time; or 3 minutes (1 round!). Speed—let's set it!

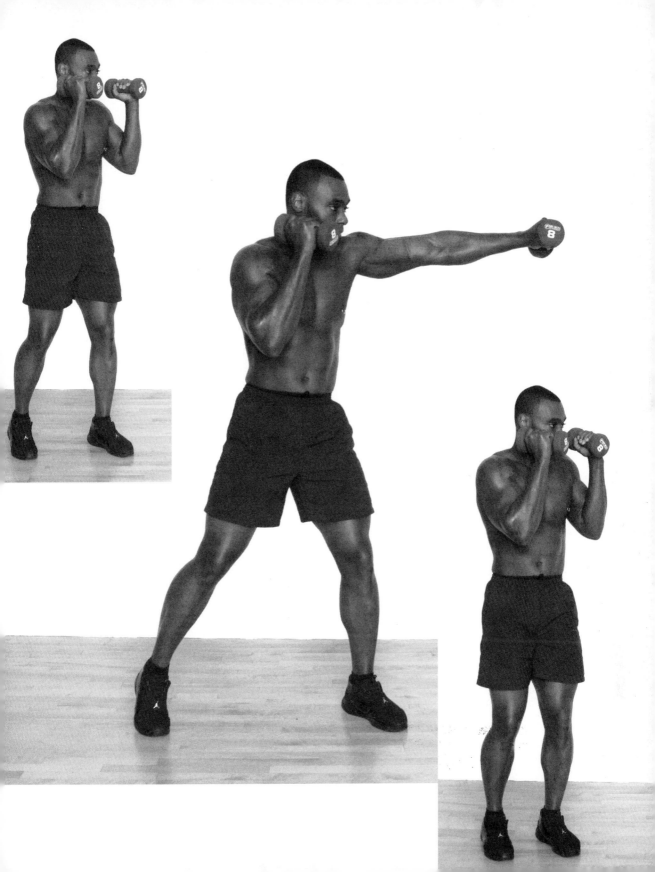

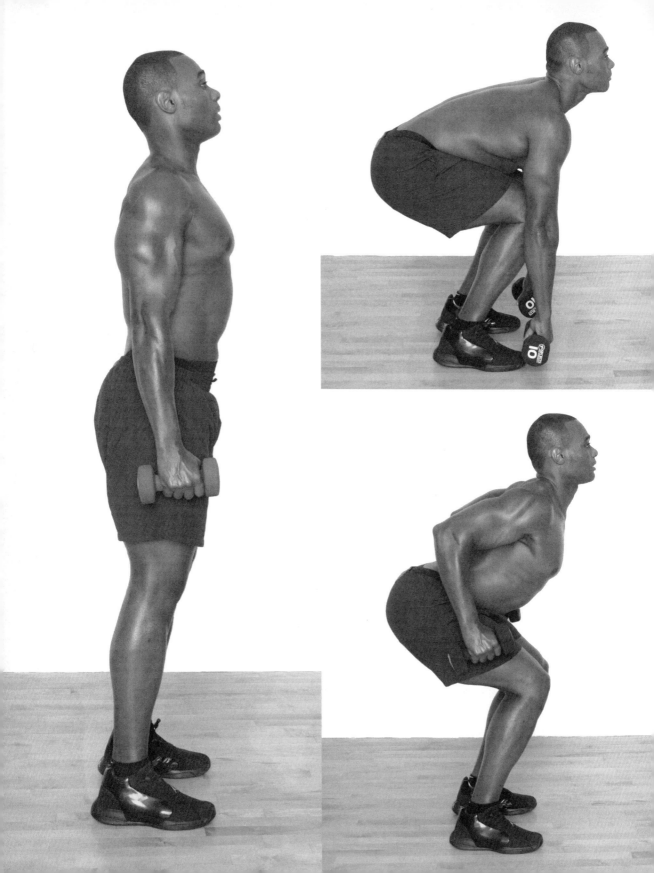

Back

You're flying blind when you train back. Curling a dumbbell, it's easy to look down and see your biceps contracting, but with rows and deadlifts, the action occurs behind you. The back's main function is to pull stuff toward you, but it takes a remarkably complicated group of muscles to do that. If you want to see all the muscles in the back, just look in a bodybuilding magazine or at an anatomy chart.

The back has more muscles than any other muscle group in the upper body. The main ones are the matching *lattisimus dorsi*, which fan out from above your waist and run up under your shoulders when viewed from the front. The back also includes a number of other muscles that, collectively, sound like dinosaurs: *teres major, teres minor, rhomboids*, and others. The back of your neck is overlaid with a muscle called the *trapezius*. Your back training somehow needs to recruit these smaller, deeper muscles. But not to worry—you got the master plan.

6. DEADLIFT ROW

WHY YOU'RE DOING IT: Although some women, in particular, shy away from this exercise, they shouldn't. Next to squatting, it's the best way to hit nearly every body part at once. In this double-barreled variation, you keep the tension on the lower back while hitting the dinosaur muscles.

HOW TO DO IT: Stand with your feet shoulder-width apart and then bend over to grasp dumbbells positioned in front of your feet, so that your knuckles face forward. Begin standing up with the dumbbells, but instead of going all the way up, as you would in a regular deadlift, stop halfway up. Instantly begin moving your elbows back to draw the dumbbells into your sides, turning your wrists as you do so that your palms face each other at belt level. Return the weights to that intermediate position, and then bend your knees to go back to the starting position. That's one full rep. Throughout, squeeze it at the top and use the lower back at the bottom.

The drill:
Three sets, 10 to 20 reps. Make it hurt!

7. REVERSE HYPEREXTENSION

WHY YOU'RE DOING IT: To help stabilize the spine, the ab muscles must work together with the muscles along the back of the spine. In most people, the abs don't carry their share of the load. They're in a weak, relaxed state for pretty much all day. This forces the back muscles to do the lion's share of spinal stabilization. No wonder 80 percent of all people will suffer back pain at some point in their life. Fortunately, the vast majority of back problems are preventable. The key is training your abs regularly and doing low-back exercises like this one. This is one of my favorite because it works the glutes as well.

HOW TO DO IT: Lie facedown on an exercise ball so that your torso and legs drape over it in a slight V formation, with your fingertips resting on the ground for support and your toes a few inches above ground. Without bending your knees, raise your legs up as high as you can without losing your stable position. Return to the starting position. Don't just do it mindlessly. Make it hurt.

The drill:
Three sets, 10 to 20 reps. Torch that lower back!

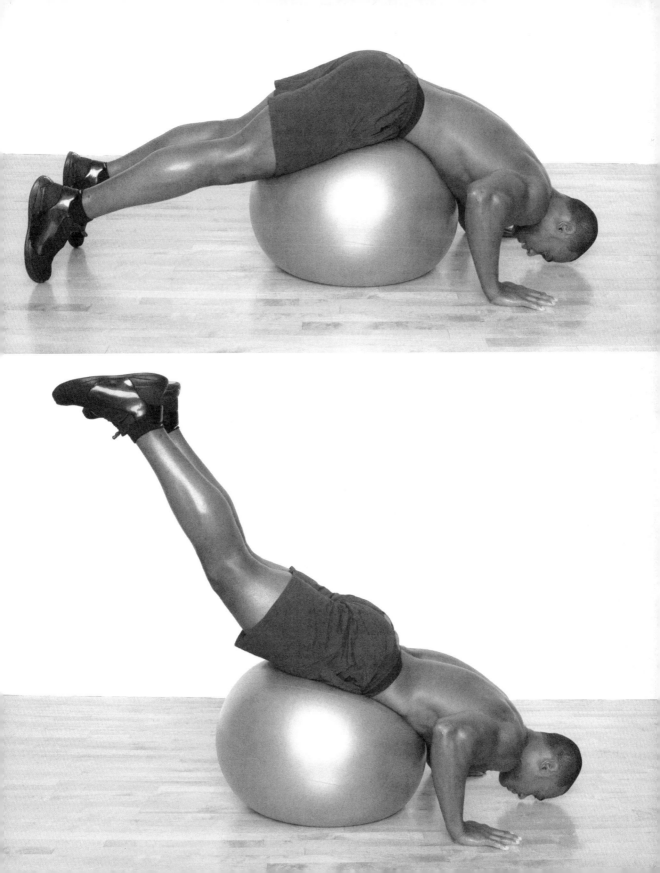

8. FOOTBALL FOOTWORK DRILL

WHY YOU'RE DOING IT: To keep your heart rate elevated. As an added bonus, this is good for developing agility.

HOW TO DO IT: Patter-step up and down in place as rapidly as possible. Picture an NFL training camp.

The drill:

Take 100 steps total. You're over 50 percent there. Do not stop! Keep it going. Almost done!

Arms

Women never used to approach me in the gym and ask, "Hey, Mark, can you show me some bicep or tricep exercises?" For that matter, they didn't inquire about upper body, period. Their preoccupations were abs, legs, and glutes. But arms? Forget it—that was a guy thing.

In the late 1980s and early 1990s, women like Angela Bassett, Angelina Jolie, and Demi Moore started showing up in movies with killer upper bodies. Ever since then, women have come up to me all the time and asked, "What's the secret to getting more tone in my arms? How can I get rid of my bat wings?" They still might be a little gun-shy about trying something like heavy barbell curls, but I explain to them that they need to lift some weight to get some tone and definition.

They also need to pay attention to their triceps (the back of the upper arm), muscles that are actually twice the size of the average biceps (the front). Most arm movements involve a combo of contraction (biceps) and extension (triceps) muscles, and for those movements to be stable, the two muscles performing them have to be balanced. Neglect one muscle in favor of the other and the machinery that normally flows smoothly gets rusty prematurely.

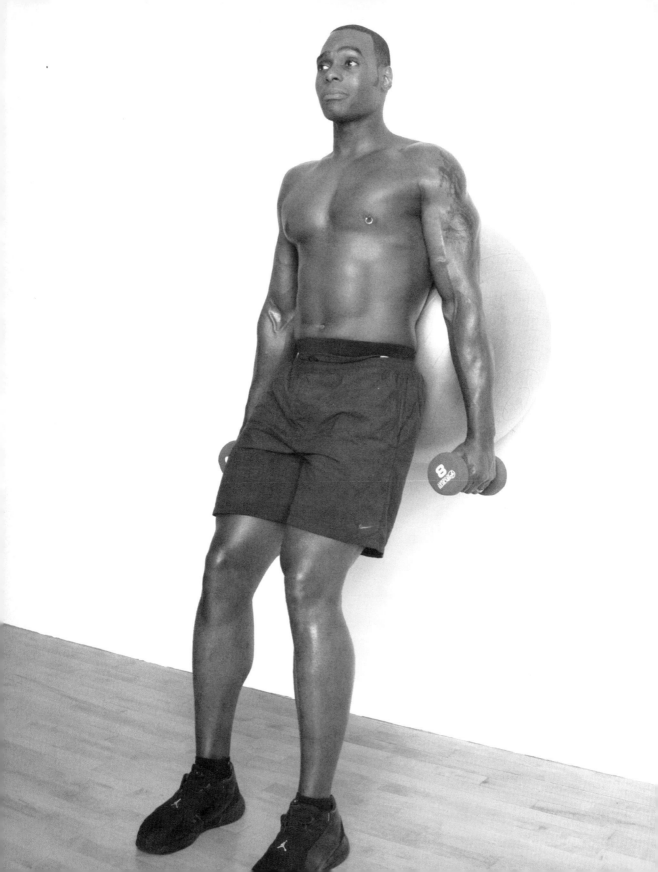

9. DUMBBELL CURL

WHY YOU'RE DOING IT: This movement is great because it's hard to cheat when performing it. You're moving one arm independently, and that insures the equal development of both arms. These bicep exercises should be done strictly without rocking or other compromises.

HOW TO DO IT: Holding a pair of dumbbells, stand with an exercise ball stuck in between your back and a wall. Hold the weights at your sides at arm's length, so that your palms are facing each other. Curl both dumbbells simultaneously toward your shoulder. As you approach the top, rotate your wrists outward so that your palm turns up. At shoulder level, give your biceps a hard squeeze and then release the weights back down slowly, rather than letting them drop. Once those dumbbells are again hanging at arm's length, immediately bang out your next repetition.

The drill:
Three sets, 15 to 30 reps. Push it out!

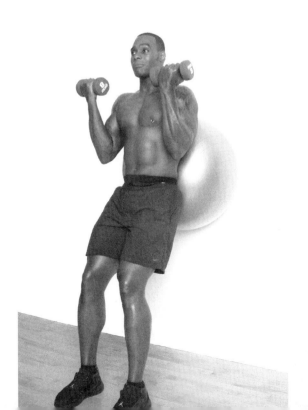

10. DUMBBELL KICKBACK

WHY YOU'RE DOING IT: Even more so than the press-down, the kickback is an isolation movement, designed to work the triceps and nothing else. That's why you don't need to use a really heavy weight; in fact, you won't be able to do so without compromising your technique, which would defeat the whole purpose of this movement.

HOW TO DO IT: Holding a dumbbell in each hand, bend at the waist until your torso is halfway between upright and parallel with the floor. Your upper arms should be pinned against your sides, with your forearms and the dumbbells hanging straight down. Slowly straighten your elbows to move the weights back, and as you arms approach full extension, rotate your wrists inward so that your palms face up. Squeeze the triceps and then bring the dumbbells back up to the starting position.

The drill:
Three sets, 15 to 30 reps.

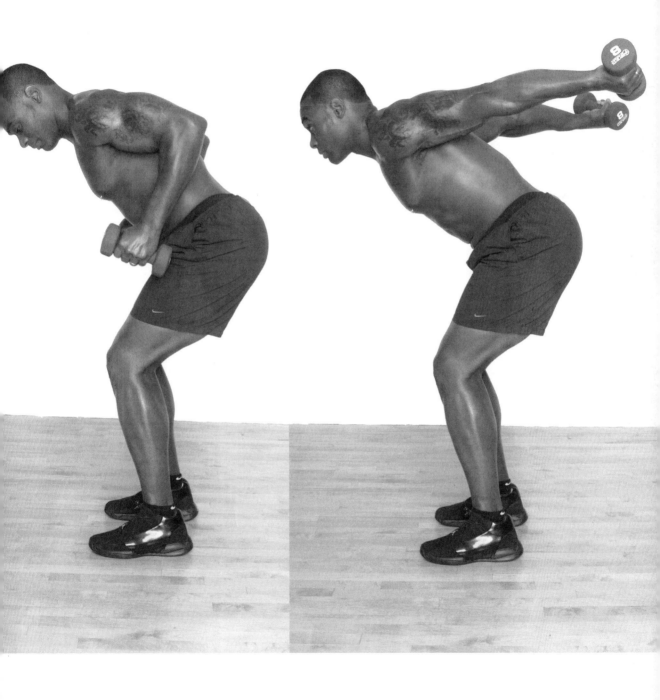

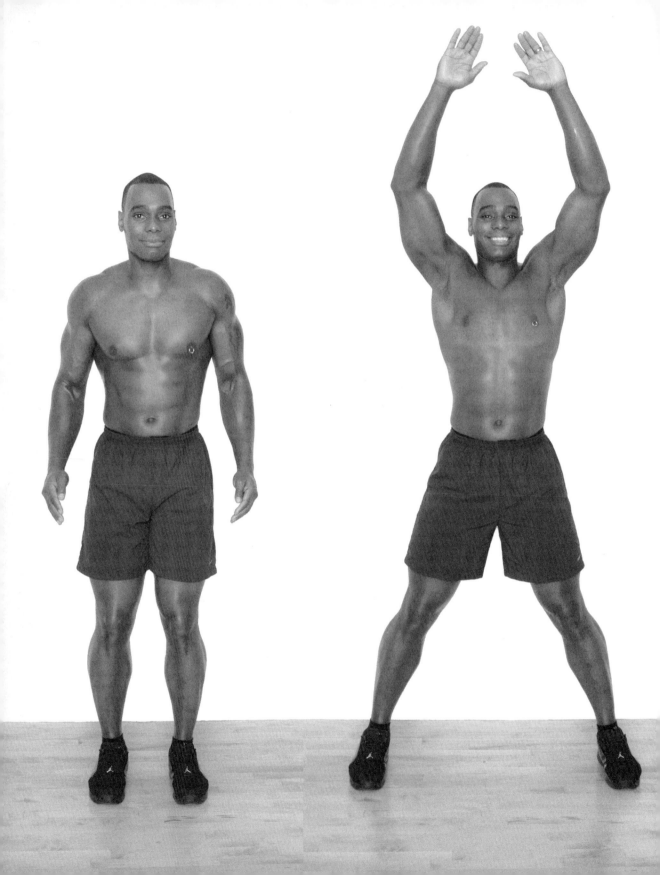

11. JUMPING JACKS

WHY YOU'RE DOING IT: Not only does this exercise keep your heart rate elevated, but it also works your calves, side delts, and small muscles of the upper thigh called adductors and abductors.

HOW TO DO IT: I know you know how to do this one! Stand with your hands at your sides and your feet together. Jump and scissor-kick your legs out to the side, simultaneously bringing your hands together above you in an arc for a clap. Return to the starting position and repeat.

The drill:

Do 100. Get busy! Count 'em out! Work your lungs.

Core

In virtually every sport, success boils down to having strong abdominals and strong lower back (the core). For you, that means that every movement you make over the course of your day involves either your stomach or your back. Everything from sitting, walking, running, and jumping to getting out of bed in the morning and picking your kids up involves your abdominals and lower back. Unfortunately, these tend to be the most overlooked body parts of all. People, you have to train your abdominals and lower back. How many people do you know with bad backs? A lot of that could have been prevented if back muscles had been strengthened to keep the stress of the joints.

Let's get crackin'. You've already worked lower back, so finish strong with abs.

12. BALL CRUNCH

WHY YOU'RE DOING IT: I'm having you do the standard crunch this way because balls are great for improving your balance, posture, body awareness, coordination, and the strength not only of your core (abs and low back) but also of the surrounding stabilizer muscles. Exercise balls increase the range of motion relative to the same ab exercises performed on the floor, ground, or workout bench. Studies have shown that a crunch performed on a ball causes your abs to work 30 percent harder than they would during a crunch performed on a rigid surface. That means fewer reps but greater results!

HOW TO DO IT: Lie face-up across an exercise ball so that the ball comfortably supports your back. Tuck your chin in slightly, focusing your eyes at a 45-degree angle—roughly the point at which ceiling meets wall. Keeping your abs contracted throughout, slowly curl your rib cage toward your hips. Hard contraction at the top, and then a slow negative to return to the starting position.

The drill:
One set, 30 to 60 reps. Hold each contraction for one second and empty those lungs.

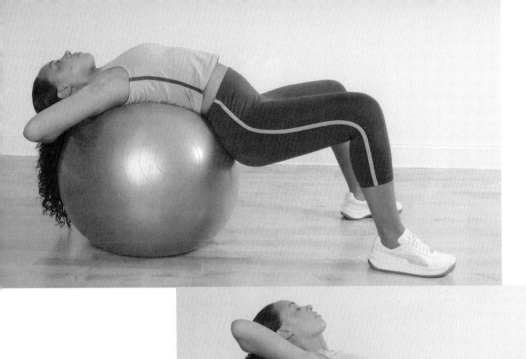

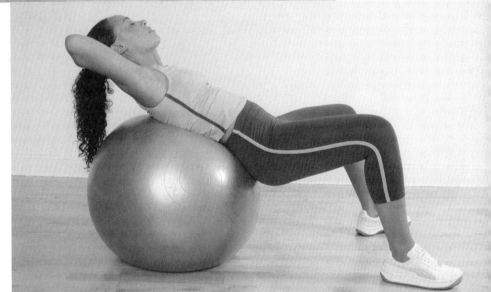

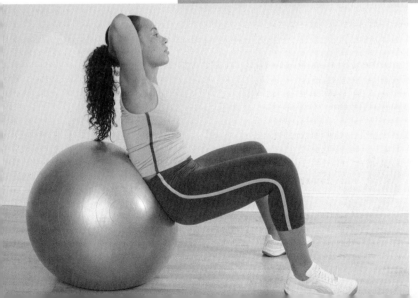

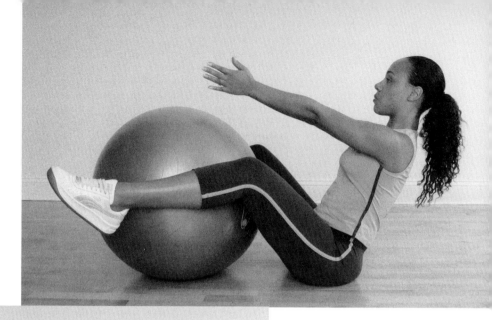

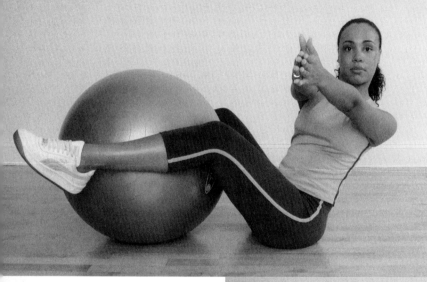

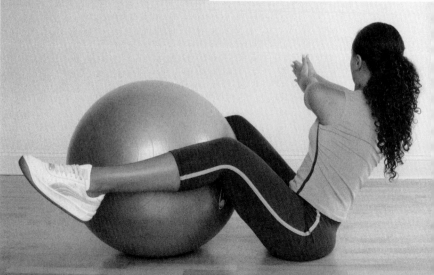

13. BALL TWIST

WHY YOU'RE DOING IT: These are designed to score a direct hit on the obliques, which run along the side of your abdominals. They have specific functions: rotating your upper body trunk and flexing it to the side. Training obliques typically involves adding a twist to exercises like the crunch and leg raise. Also, the sides of the abdominals are a key attribute of a hip-hop hard body. LL and D'Angelo have great obliques, and it separates them from the rest!

HOW TO DO IT: Sit with your butt on the floor, squeezing an exercise ball between your legs. Lean back slightly, extend both arms out in front of you, and clasp your hands together. Keeping your legs stationary and your arms straight, rotate your torso as far as you can in one direction, and then reverse it until you've reached the end of your range of motion in the other direction. Continue going side to side until you finish the set. The more it burns, the harder you push! Slow and controlled.

The drill:
One set, 30 to 60 reps.

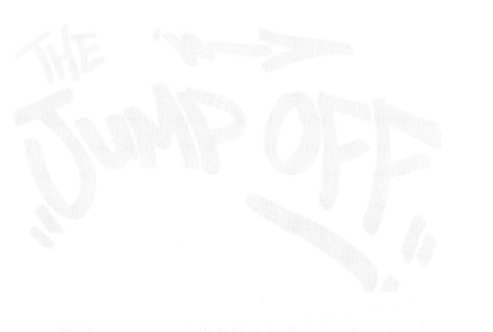

14. BALL TUCK

WHY YOU'RE DOING IT: You shouldn't overlook exercises that emphasize the lower half of the abdominal wall, and this is a great one that won't ever let you overlook them again.

HOW TO DO IT: Assume a push-up position and place your feet up on an exercise ball. Keeping your upper body stationary, use your feet to roll the ball in toward your torso. Extend your legs back out to return to the starting position.

The drill:

One set, 30 reps. Squeeze and release slowly. Show me you want it!

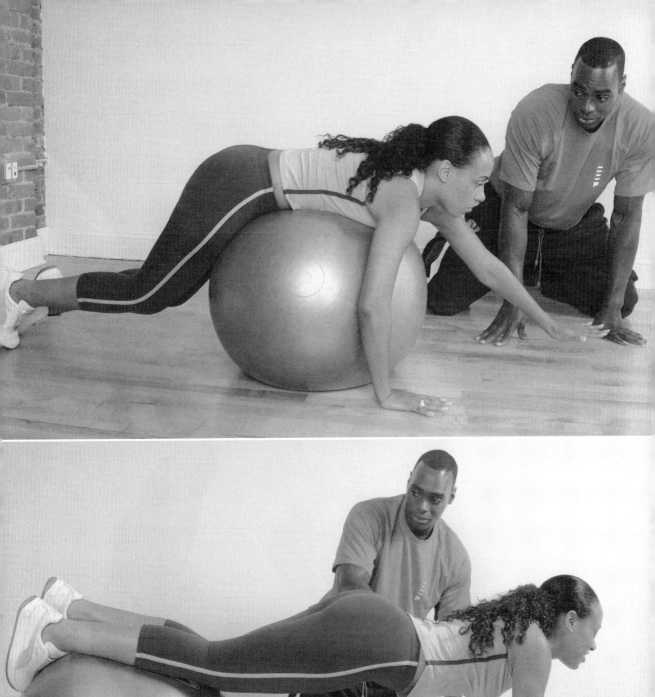
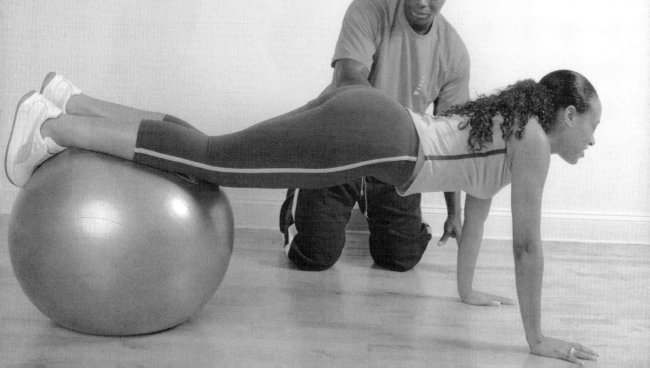

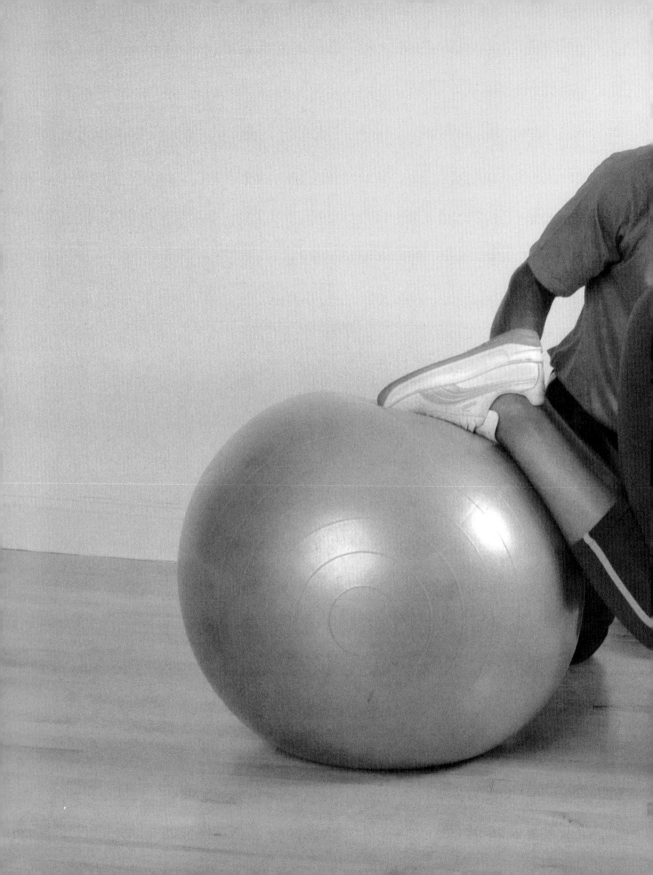

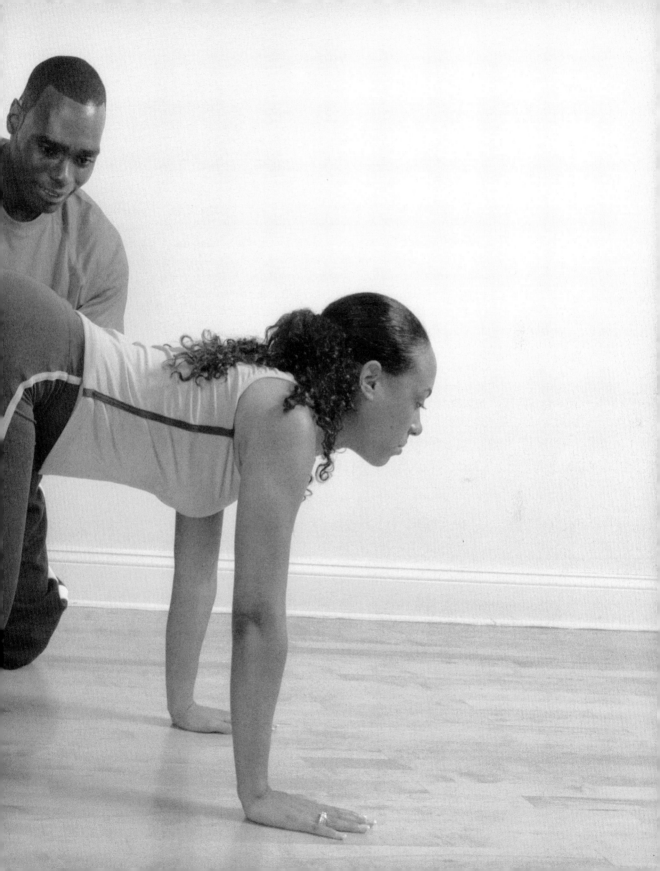

How to Get Arms Like Busta Rhymes

Buss-a-buss is extremely charismatic! When I train him, the other people working out are like, "Hey, Busta, wass' up, man?" Even old ladies come up and talk to him because he doesn't send off that unapproachable vibe. He's a really likable guy and he feeds off the energy of people training around him. I haven't really noticed that with any other artist I've trained.

But don't get it twisted—he goes right for the jugular when it comes time to training. Busta also has a great capacity for flicking the switch when the time comes to work hard. You don't have to bust his ass. He *wants* to push it. He *wants* to feel some pain. So you definitely know that he came to the right person. When we first hooked up, he had some body fat stored around his waist and midsection, but his arms were very lean. The problem was, he didn't have much muscle on them, nor did he have much separation between the biceps and the triceps. Because he has a long, lanky frame, we set out to put some size on him. My strategy with him was to stick with basic movements like barbell curls and hit it heavy. We also got his guns looking crazy by resting only 30 seconds between sets, allowing him to completely exhaust his biceps.

Busta Rhymes: Six weeks into his transformation and down 25 pounds.

Here's how you can achieve the same look. Start off doing two sets, 15 reps apiece, of lying cable curls. To do them, lie on the floor with your feet against the weight stack. Hold a handle attached to the low cable pulley at arm's length. From there, just do your curls horizontally. These are great because your back is stabilized and you can't cheat by rocking on the upstroke.

Next, bang out the same amount of incline dumbbell curls. Raise the weight up a quarter of the way, take it back down, and then lift it all the way back up to your shoulder—that equals one rep! Wrap it up with seated concentration curls. Same drill as the other two moves: two sets, 15 reps.

On all bicep moves, don't hesitate to change the speed at which you raise and lower the weight. Going slower than normal is one of the best-kept secrets for stressing the muscle fibers in your biceps and making them grow. But don't go slow all the time. The idea is to train your neuromuscular system differently. Also, make sure that you control the weight, rather than letting the weight control you. Flex your biceps first and let the contraction move the weight.

Last but not least, don't let your biceps outgrow your triceps, or vice versa. An imbalance can make you vulnerable to injury, just like weak abs can lead to a back injury.

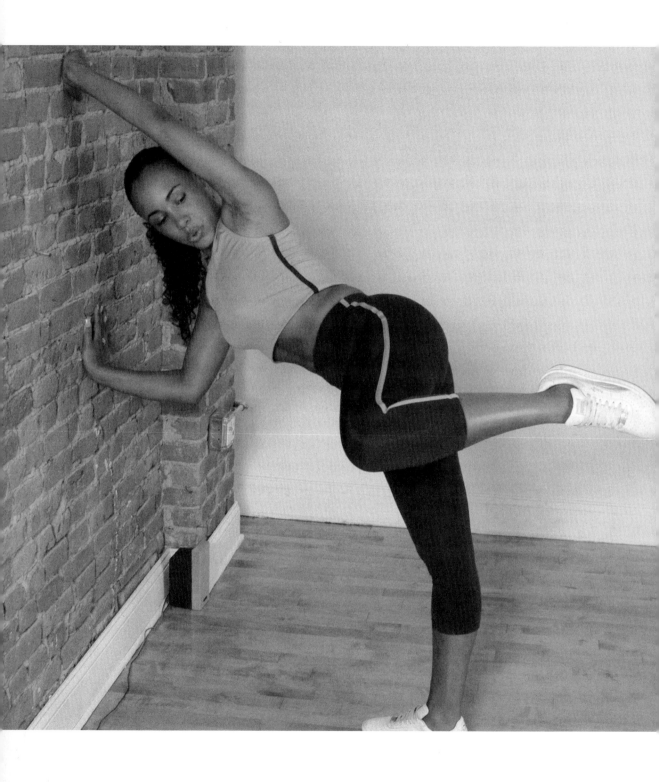

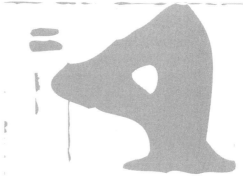

The Lower-Body Attack

I wish I had a dime for every time women have told me that they don't want to train their legs with weights because, "It'll bulk me up and make me less flexible." In the next breath these same women will say, "But I want to get toned!" Let me set you straight. If you don't have some muscle, there is nothing to define. But women don't have enough testosterone flowing naturally in their bodies to develop excessive leg musculature. Even women who <u>want</u> to get huge, freaky legs like bodybuilders can only achieve that look through a fanatical effort that includes taking synthetic hormones. (They get big muscles, but they also start to sound like

Darth Vader and grow beards. Something to avoid.) But Mary J. goes all-out during big leg day, and look at her wheels—toned but very feminine. This is the definition you want, and you need to build muscle to get it.

Then there are the guys. For them, it's all about the "beach muscles," bigger chest, tri's and bi's. I can hear you now, Playboy: "Mark, I usually wear jeans so why should I waste time training a part of my body that no one's going to see anyway?" Newsflash: legs make up more than 50 percent of your body, and when was the last time you wore long pants at the beach anyway? Beyond appearance, you need strong legs to carry yourself around. As for flexibility, training with weights will improve that, not rob you of it. Olympic weight lifters are among the world's most flexible athletes.

What men and women are willing to do for legs, ironically, is hours of slow, repetitive cardio on the exercise bike, treadmill, and stair climber. That'll help build your endurance, but it won't do much for the shape of your wheels. If you don't believe me, watch a track-and-field event on TV. First, check out the stick legs of the long-distance runners, whose training consists of endless hours of cardio work. Next, scope out the sprinters, with their tight leg muscles and rounded glutes. In terms of building your body, the advantages of resistance training over cardio are plain to see.

I've designed this second session to work your entire lower body, from your glutes all the way down to your calves. Like the other two workouts, it's a double whammy, a two-for-one special: cardio and weights together, nonstop-till-you-drop action. We're going to expand your lung capacity while building your muscles and burning fat. In fact, you burn more calories training legs than any other body part.

The same three rules that go for the upper-body workout apply here as well: Always warm up your muscles before training; stretch after warm-up and during and after training; and keep up the tempo. *Do not stop to rest*. After you finish one body part, take a few sips of water, stretch, and move on to your next set or exercise. The more it hurts, the harder you attack. The harder it goes, the harder you go. Less rest between sets means more results for you.

Are you with me?

It's your body—you can do it! This will work for you, so have faith! Don't let a little pain stand between you and your wheels of steel.

The Lower-Body Workout

EXERCISE	SETS	REPS/TIME
Quads and Hamstrings		
1. Jump rope	1	5 minutes or 300 skips (This is designed to warm you up as much as it is to work these body parts.)
2. Ball squat	3	15–30 reps
3. Speed jabs	3	15–20 reps per leg
4. Reverse lunge	1	100 jabs each arm, 20 at a time; or 3 minutes (1 round! Speed, baby! Pump that jab! Fight for the new you!)
Hamstrings and Glutes		
5. Knee-ups	1	100 reps per leg, 20 at a time
6. Stiff-legged deadlift	3	10–20 reps (Stretch those hammies!)
7. Ball leg curl	3	10–20 reps (Hold and squeeze.)
8. Pulsing squat	1	30 reps (Chest out; no hunching over.)
9. Glute squeeze	1	30 reps
Calves (You should be hurting by now, but keep going!)		
10. Speed drill	1	100 steps
11. Standing calf raise	1	30 reps
12. Kneeling calf raise	1	30 reps
Abs (Almost done! Finish strong.)		
13. Pick one from ab grid, Column A	1	30
14. Pick one from ab grid, Column B	1	30
15. Pick one from ab grid, Column C	1	30 per side

Quads and Hamstrings

1. JUMPING ROPE

WHY YOU'RE DOING IT: Get your heart rate elevated, expand your lung capacity, and improve your speed and agility. It'll also warm up your body for the workout to follow.

HOW TO DO IT: See Chapter 3, which also included this exercise. Keep your feet low to the ground. If you mess up halfway through, keep going! Everybody messes up. It's the champions that keep going. Your heart isn't worried about your form. Work it!

Now that's what I'm talkin' about. I knew you could do it!

The drill:
Five minutes, or 300 skips.

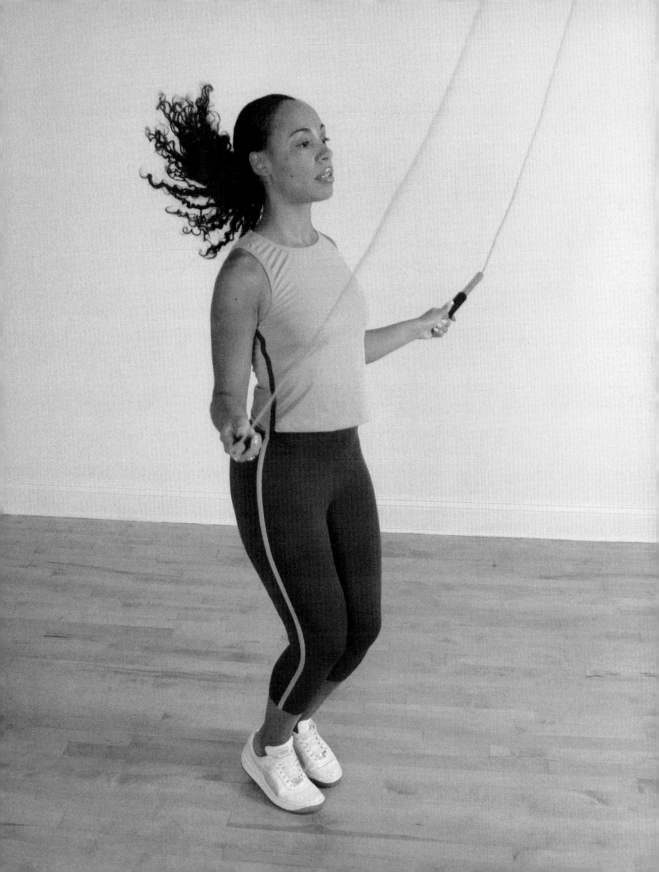

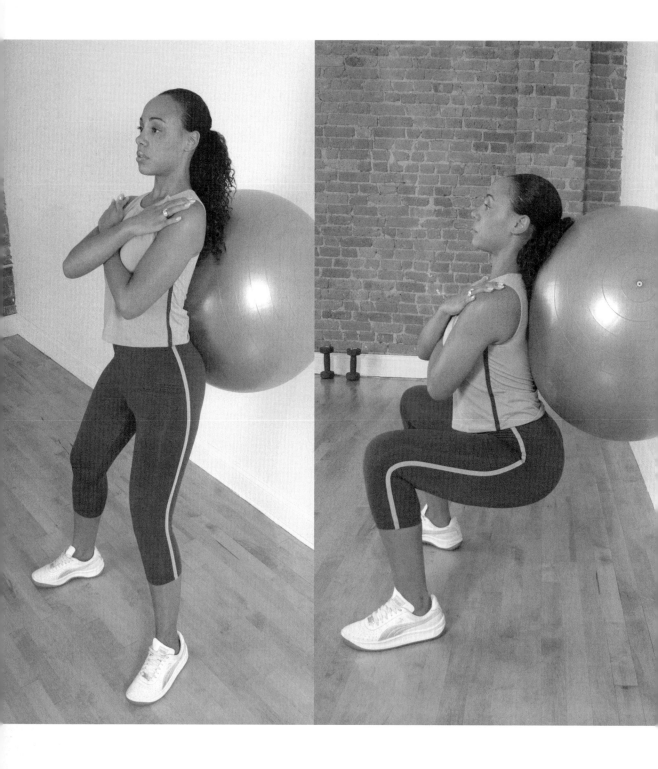

2. BALL SQUAT

WHY YOU'RE DOING IT: The squat is the king of all lower-body exercises. Done correctly, it works the glutes, quads, and hamstrings all in one shot. By squatting with a ball against your back, you ensure proper form. Controlling the ball also works your stabilization muscles. If you really work this exercise, you are going to win.

HOW TO DO IT: Stand up straight with an exercise ball between your back and the wall. Your feet should be slightly wider than shoulder-width apart, your feet angled out slightly, arms crossed over your chest. Looking straight ahead, bend your knees and drop your hips back and down, "rolling" against the ball until your thighs are parallel to the floor or slightly lower. Keep the tension on the legs. Don't bounce at the bottom, but don't stop, either. Drive up to return to the starting position.

To challenge yourself more, hold a dumbbell between your legs with both hands while you're doing it.

The drill:
Three sets, 15 to 30 reps.

3. REVERSE LUNGES

WHY YOU'RE DOING IT: This is a great exercise to get you looking right from behind.

HOW TO DO IT: Stand holding a dumbbell in each hand. Take a step back with one foot and bend that knee to lower your torso until your front thigh is parallel with the ground and your rear leg trails behind. Use your glutes and hamstrings. Keeping your hips and shoulders squared to the front and your abs tight, exhale as you push off your lead leg to return to the starting position. Push. *Push!* See your legs getting tighter and stronger in your mind as you train.

Repeat for the desired number of reps, then switch leg positions and do an identical number of reps.

The drill:
Three sets, 10 to 20 reps per leg; 20 to 40 reps total per set.

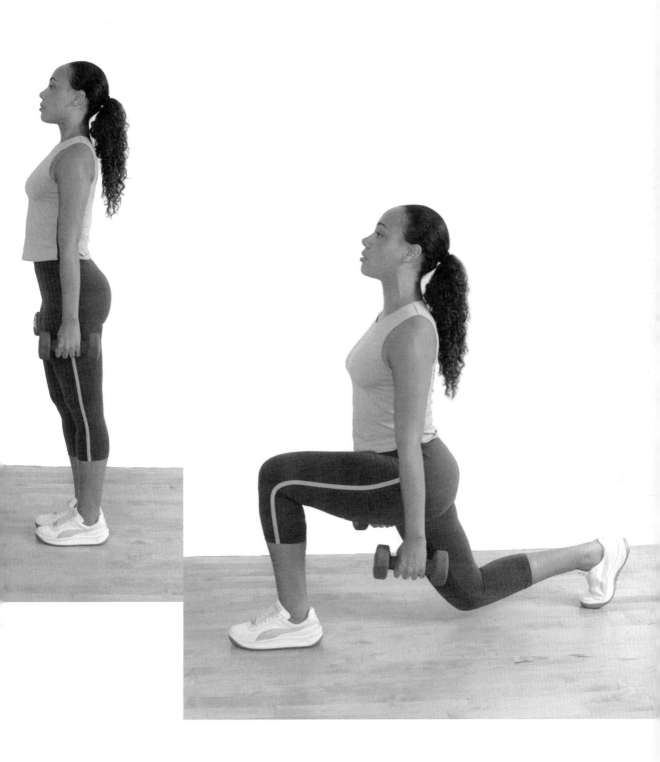

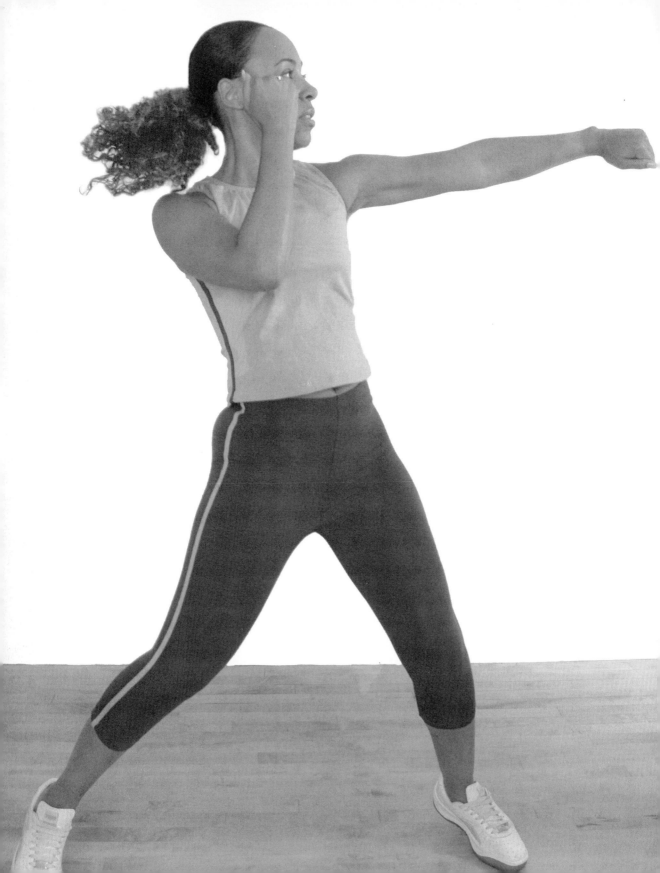

WHY YOU'RE DOING IT: Your legs are on fire but you've got to work the heart now. Tap into those fat stores. That's what it's all about. Remember, this is your body. Don't give up! *Dig!*

HOW TO DO IT: Stay on the balls of your feet and extend your elbows to throw rapid-fire punches. Punch as you step. Keep your feet moving through-out. It's all about speed. Step with the left leg, jab with the left arm for 50, then do the same number on the right. You're so hard-core on this one.

The drill:
100 jabs each arm, 20 at a time; or 3 minutes (1 round!).

Glutes and Hamstrings

No body part comes in as many shapes and sizes as the glutes, known more affectionately as cheeks, bottom, cakes, butt, rear, or—my personal favorite—derriere. Everyone appreciates a nice backyard. Whole exercise books and dozens of infomercials have been dedicated to this body part. But you don't need to train it (or them) for an hour to get results. All you have to do is really concentrate when you train and really squeeze the muscles you're attacking. You can make one set feel like 100 reps if you go slow and really squeeze it. It's all about quality.

Your glutes actually consist of three muscles: the *gluteus maximus*, the *gluteus minimus*, and the *gluteus medius*. The latter two are largely obscured from view; the maximus is the one you're checking out on rap videos. Glutes do more than just draw stares, however; they're also integral to basic aspects of posture and movement, such as standing erect and walking. And when it's time to lift things, the glutes—along with the low back, abs, quads, and hamstrings—become the primary center of power for your body.

Okay, time to kick glutes.

5. KNEE-UPS

WHY YOU'RE DOING IT: This is another aerobic interval exercise to keep your heart pumping and fat burning. Q-Tip loves this one.

HOW TO DO IT: Stand up straight and kick one of your knees up as high as you can. *Attack.* Return to the starting position and repeat. Keep your arms swinging in rhythm with the kicks. Opposite arm, opposite leg. Higher—higher! Get it up! Knees above the belly button. Drive that right knee up 20 times, and without rest, jump on the left knee. Keep going until you hit a buck—100, baby.

The drill:

Do 20 kicks with one leg, and then 20 with another, until you've done 100 reps with each. Switching back and forth is important, which is why I don't like a lot of workouts I see on video or read in books! Doing 50 or 60 kicks at a time with one leg will open you up to an overuse injury, and an injury will take us out of the season. Safety first!

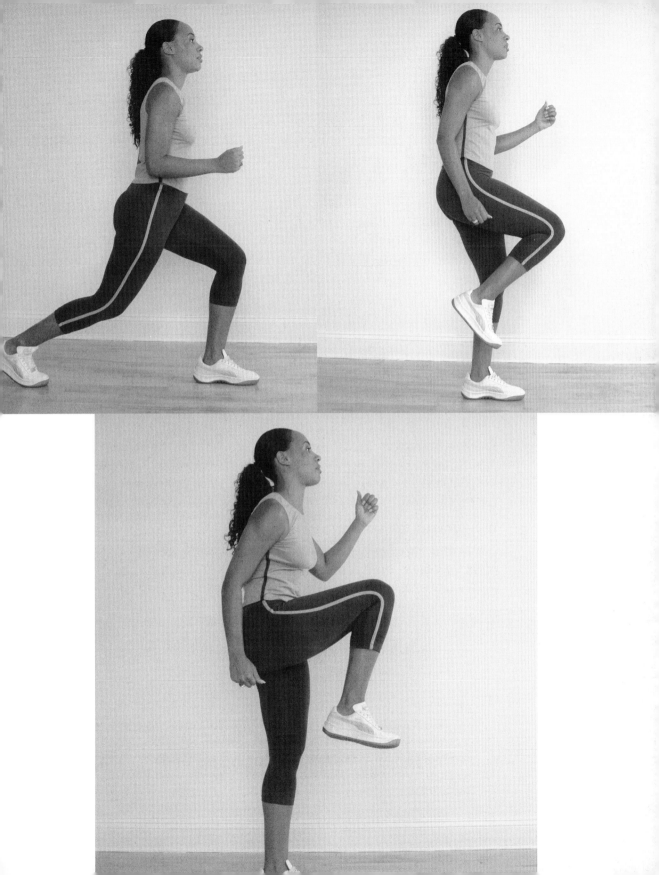

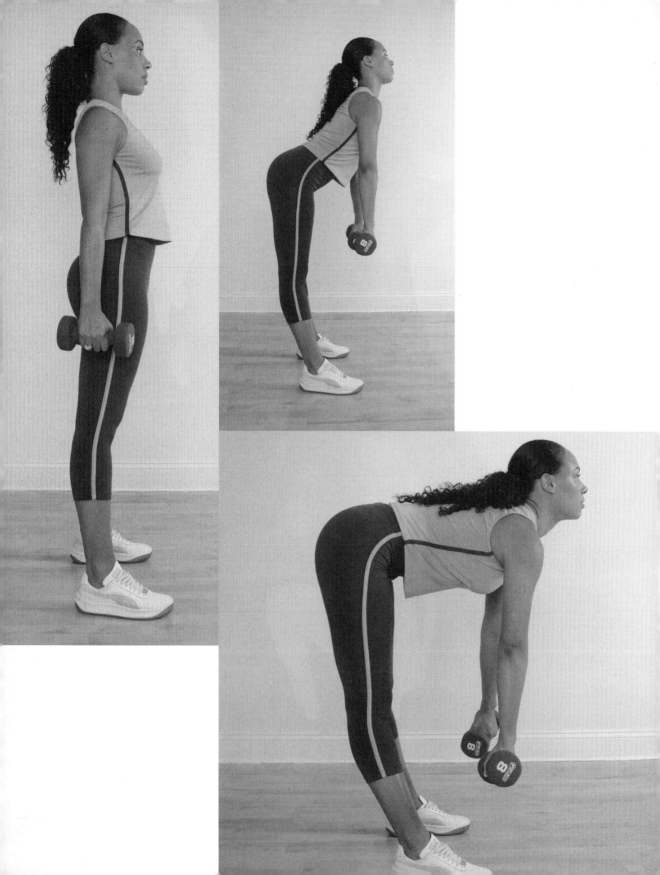

6. STIFF-LEGGED DEADLIFT

WHY YOU'RE DOING IT: To give those hamstrings a good stretch under resistance before you get to the burnin' leg curl that comes next. My female clients swear by this exercise.

HOW TO DO IT: Stand holding dumbbells at arm's length, palms facing each other. With your chest out, bend at the waist and drop your hips back, feeling the pull in your hamstrings. Go down as far as you can without curving your back, rotating your wrists so that your palms face behind you at the bottom. Come back up slowly, pulling with the hamstrings and squeezing the glutes.

The drill:

Three sets, 10 to 20 reps.

7. BALL LEG CURL

WHY YOU'RE DOING IT: To blast those hamstrings and etch in that detail for a truly hard body!

HOW TO DO IT: Lie face-up with your feet elevated on an exercise ball. Use your heels to pull the ball toward you, lifting your hips off the ground as you bend your knees. It's all about feeling the hamstrings throughout the entire motion. When your hips are fully extended and you can't bring the ball any closer, reverse the movement to return slowly to the starting position.

Stretch, drink, and continue the attack.

The drill:
Three sets, 10 to 20 reps.

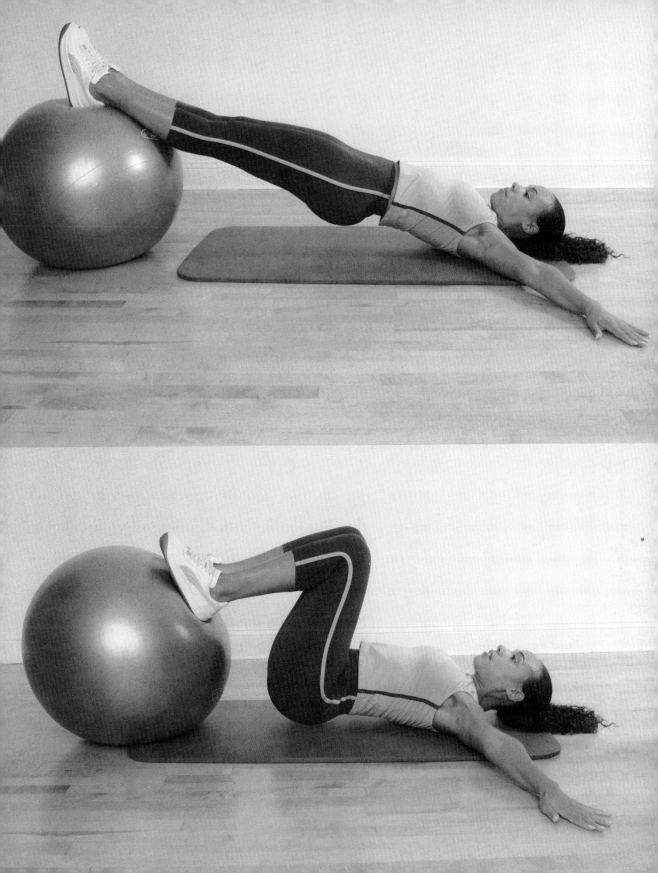

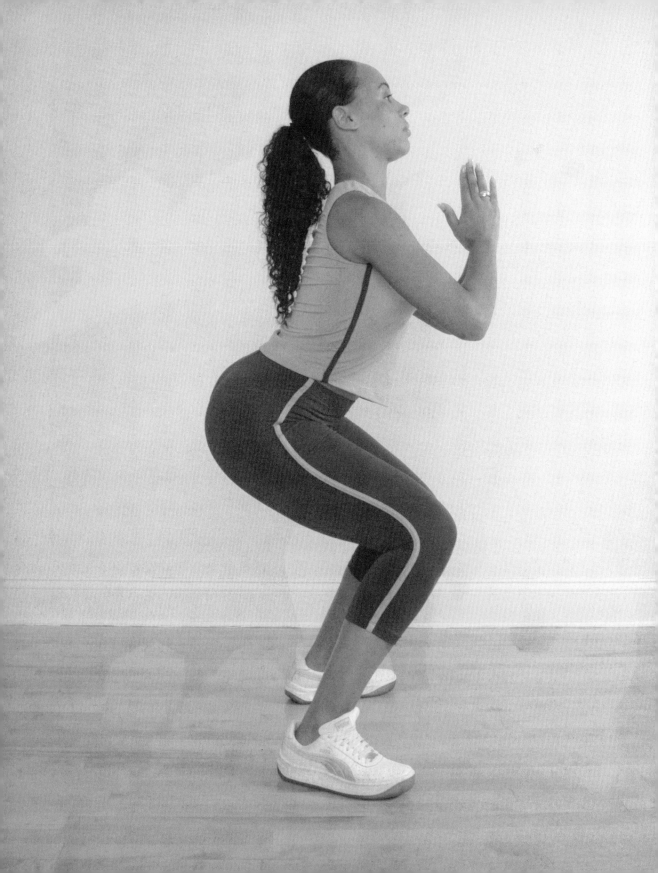

8. PULSING SQUAT

WHY YOU'RE DOING IT: This is where your glutes are activated the most. Trust me—you'll feel the burn back there.

HOW TO DO IT: Stand up straight with your feet slightly wider than shoulder-width apart, toes angled out slightly. Your hands should be pressed together in front of your breastbone as if you're meditating. Looking straight ahead, bend your knees and drop your hips back and down until your thighs are parallel to the floor or slightly lower. Keep your chest out. Push through your heels to rise back up, but stop after a few inches and go right back down. Continue doing these "partials" rapid-fire until you've completed the desired number of reps. *Push!*

If you want to add resistance, hold a dumbbell between your legs with both hands.

The drill:
One set, 30 reps. It's only one set—attack! Do not rest until you hit 30!

9. GLUTE SQUEEZE

WHY YOU'RE DOING IT: More glute work. Everyone wears jeans, right? It's your body—shape it into what you want it to be.

HOW TO DO IT: Lie with your shoulder blades resting on an exercise ball, your arms across your chest, and your feet planted on the ground so that your knees are bent and your thighs are nearly vertical. Squeeze your glutes hard to raise your hips as high as you can. This will cause your shoulder blades to roll up the ball a few inches. Take one second at the top for the contraction. Squeeze as hard as you can! Lower your hips back to the starting position.

The drill:

One set, 30 reps. This is not a typo! One set, 30 reps!

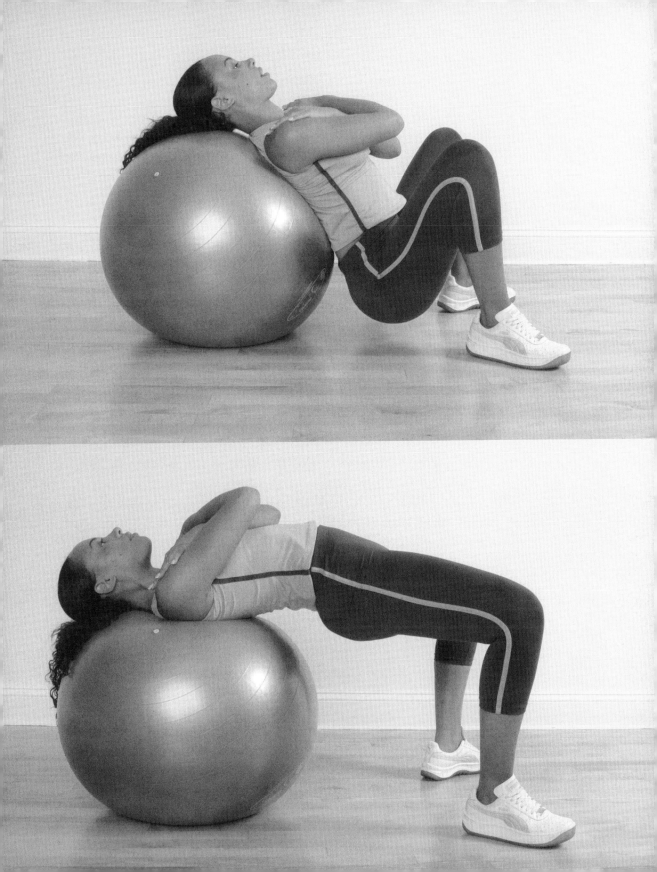

Calves

Diamonds are indeed a girl's best friend, and that applies to diamond-cut calves, too. Nothing looks better than a pair of sculpted calves above sexy high heels. Nor should guys ignore this important body part. It's important for the beach as well as for the vertical jump when you're playing ball.

To understand how to train calves, let me give you a quick anatomy lesson. The calf comprises two primary muscles: the *soleus* and the *gastrocnemius*. Unlike the soleus, which doesn't cross the knee joint, the gastroc actually crosses both the ankle and knee joints. In fact, it assists in flexing (bending) your knee and helps prevent your knee joint from being hyperextended. Because it serves these additional functions in a bent-knee position, the gastroc becomes less involved in raising your heel than it does when your leg is straight. So when you're cranking out endless sets of seated calf raises, you're hammering your soleus, the workhorse of the calf, but you're not doing a particularly effective job of recruiting the gastroc.

Today, we'll hit both.

10. SPEED DRILL

WHY YOU'RE DOING IT: You know what time it is. Gotta get that heart rate up and activate those calves!

HOW TO DO IT: Run in place as hard as you can. Get those knees above your belly button. Keep your arms moving. *Faster.* Dig, dig, *dig!*

The drill:
One hundred steps. Climb that mountain. Get that hard body!

11. STANDING CALF RAISE

WHY YOU'RE DOING IT: No calf workout is complete without a standing exercise, because only from an upright position can you really zero in on the gastrocnemius.

HOW TO DO IT: Stand on the floor or, better, on a step so that the edge rests between your toes and the balls of your feet. Keeping your legs straight and your torso erect, lower your heels as far as you can. Push off the balls of your feet until you're almost on tiptoes. This can also be done one leg at a time.

The drill:

One set, 30 reps.

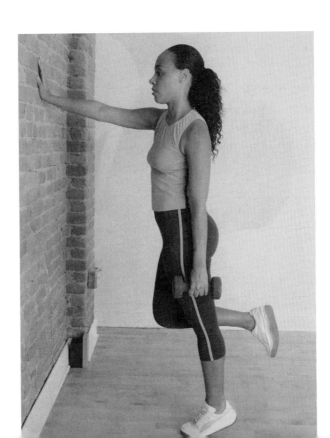

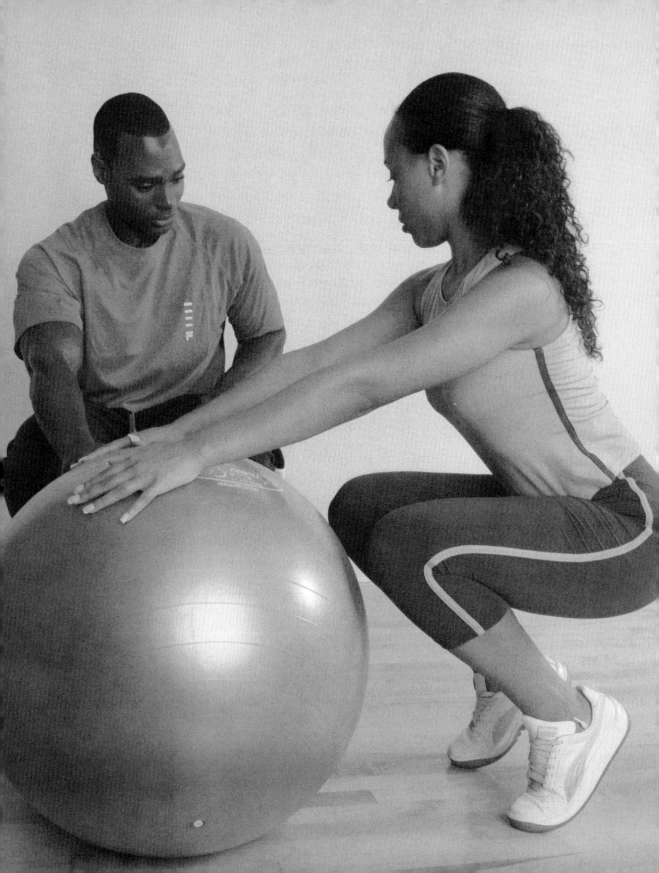

12. KNEELING CALF RAISE

WHY YOU'RE DOING IT: This exercise targets your soleus muscle for complete development.

HOW TO DO IT: Squat in front of an exercise ball so that your feet are flat on the floor and your thighs are parallel with the same. Place your hands on top of the ball. Push off the balls of your feet to raise your knees as high as you can, and then go back down to the starting position. *Feel* the calves. Work it.

The drill:

One set, 30 reps. Burn, baby, burn! You should be cursing me by now, but just think about the results.

Abdominals

WHY YOU'RE DOING IT: You're doing abs again because they're endurance muscles—they contract frequently and must remain that way for long periods of time. The "grid" concept below is designed to ensure that you achieve complete, balanced development throughout your midsection, rather than just strong upper abs from a constant diet of traditional crunches.

HOW TO DO IT: Pick one exercise from group A, B, and C and do one set of 30 (per side for obliques). You know the drill: sip some water, stretch, and then move onto an exercise from the next group. The bottom three movements are more advanced.

Do not rest—finish strong!

A: UPPER ABs

Ball Crunch
See description from upper-body workout.

Ball Extension
Rest your forearms on top of an exercise ball, your elbows tucked into your sides and your legs straight, with your feet spread apart. Roll the ball forward on your forearms, taking your elbows slightly away from your body, and then pull the ball back in.

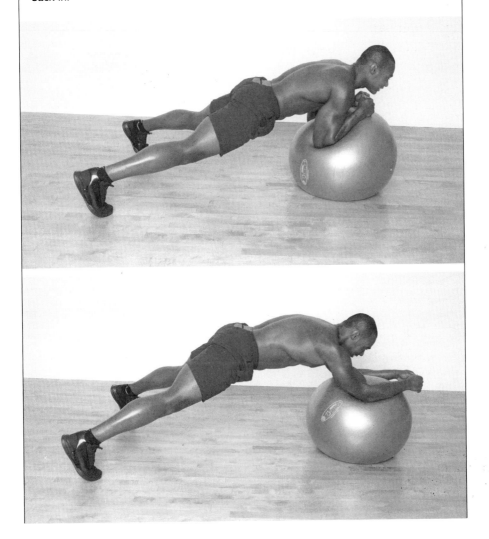

Full-Body Crunch
Lie on the floor with your back on a mat, your hands behind your head and your legs hovering over the floor, knees slightly bent. Crunch your torso toward your pelvis as you simultaneously draw your knees in toward your chest.

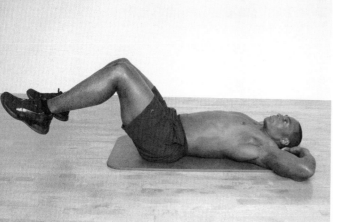
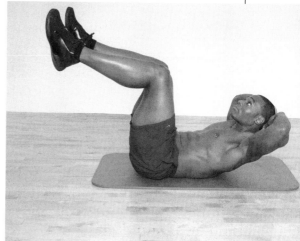

B: LOWER ABs

Ball Tuck
See description from upper-body workout.

Reverse Crunch (not pictured)
Lie on the floor with your back on a mat, your hands behind your head and your legs hovering over the floor, knees slightly bent. Keeping your head and torso fixed, bring your knees in toward your chest.

Hanging Leg Raise (not pictured)
Hang from a bar or support using a shoulder-width, overhand grip. Bend your knees so that they form 90-degree angles. Rotate your hips forward and bring your knees up as close to your chest as possible. Lower your knees back to where your thighs are parallel to the ground.

C: OBLIQUES

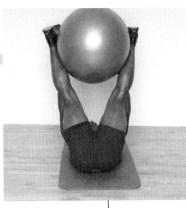

Ball Twist
See description from upper-body workout.

Ball Rotation
Lie flat on your back with an exercise ball between your legs, which should be raised perpendicular to your torso and the floor. Keeping your upper body fixed, roll the ball by rotating your legs from one side to the other, going as far as you can in each direction.

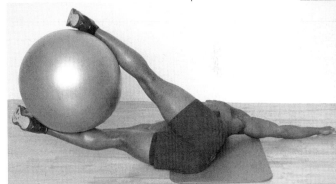

Ball Jackknife
Lean back on a ball with your right hand behind your neck, your left arm draped over the ball, and your feet planted. Your left leg should be straight and your right knee bent. Take your left leg and crunch it toward your right elbow. Do 10 each side and then switch, alternating until you complete 30 reps a side.
LL loves this one—very tough!

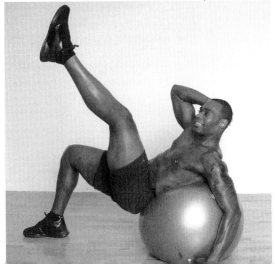

How to Get Legs Like Mary J. Blige

No one can teach you to sing like Mary J. Blige—that's one in a million. But you can get legs like hers, and I should know. I helped her sculpt them.

Her wheels weren't always off the hook, mind you. As I mention elsewhere, when Mary and I first hooked up, she had fired two other trainers. More than likely they weren't producing results, and Mary is all about the bottom line. When I joined her team, my job was to produce the same sort of results she gets in the studio. Legs posed a particular challenge for us. Like a lot of sisters, Mary is naturally bottom-heavy, so my whole thing was balance, because her upper body was a lot smaller than her lower body. That made her look hippier than she actually was. So the goal became to tone down her size below the waist while toning up her leg muscles and building her upper body. We did that using a combination of squats, using relatively heavy weights and high reps, and uphill sprinting. You can get the same results by dedicating an extra session each week just to legs.

Here's how: Begin this special leg workout with 10 sets of squats. You'll curse me when you're doing them, but the thanks will come later. You don't have to use much weight—in fact, you don't have to use any weight at first while you become acclimated to holding the bar across your shoulders—but you need this high volume to really sculpt your legs and butt.

Next, do either uphill sprints or double-leg bounding, where you jump in the air repeatedly, switching a scissors-stance foot position each time. Three sets of 10 reps should do the trick here. Then come some stiff-legged deadlifts, for hamstrings, and pulsing squats, to finish off the entire glute and upper-leg complex.

If you're worried about your glutes getting too big from all that leg training, you have nothing to fear—just so long as you follow the diet in **Chapter 7**. That's the key thing that people mess up on. They might be good with the weights, but they don't diet. So they get bigger and then blame it on the weights. If you're eating right, rather than your butt gettin' too big, you should see a reconfiguration, with fat vanishing and muscle moving into all the right places. You should also see people start to notice your new hard body!

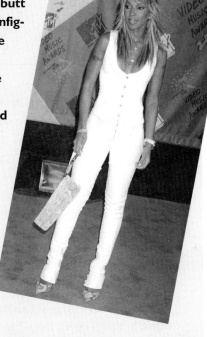

I've given you the approach I used with Mary, but be open-minded. Experiment. Find out what works best for you. You can read a million routines in magazines, but you won't know what works until you've tried different things. Mary's legs were a problem area, but now she's known for them. You can achieve the same transformation only if you expect nothing less!

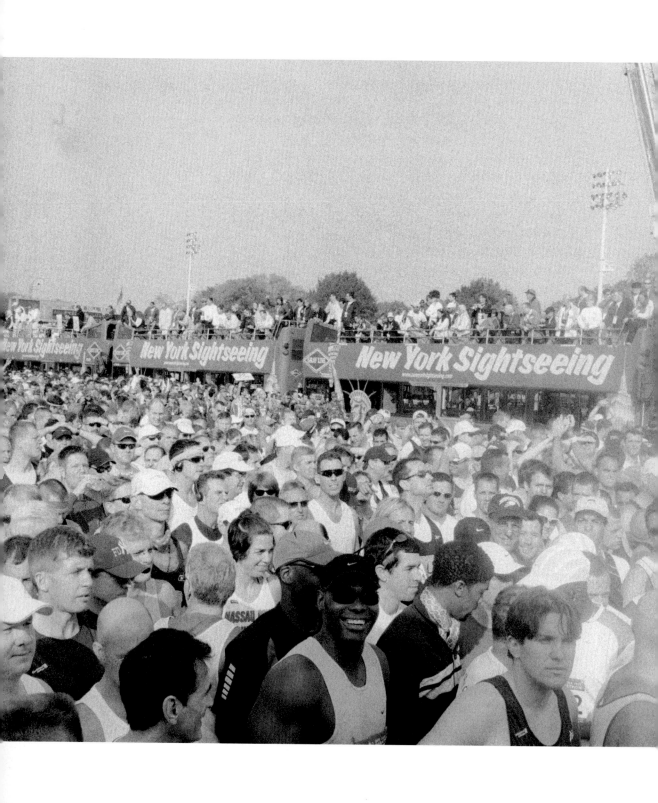

Outside the Box—The Outdoor Workout

You might do a double take if you see a guy running through the park with a parachute behind his back. But the fact that I use such an unorthodox piece of equipment reflects two fundamental truths about my training style: I love the hard-core drills, and I love workin' it outdoors. There's just something about getting outside, moving around in nature, and breaking a sweat while soaking up some rays that makes you feel alive.

The simplicity of outdoor training really appeals to me. Simplicity characterizes the indoor workouts, which can be done as easily at home as in the gym. But the outdoor session is a no-brainer. All you need to do is put on some clothes and step outside. The only thing you must have is oxygen, and Mother Nature delivers all of that for free.

This workout is about more than just having some fun in the sun, although I want you to have a good time while you're doing it. Outdoor training forces your muscles and cardiorespiratory system to become functional in the real world. I've met a lot of dudes who can push a ton of iron in the gym, and a lot of women who can sit on a recumbent bike for hours, but make them run two city blocks, and they act like they're on the verge of collapse. That's why I'm really proud of what Puffy accomplished in the New York City Marathon. Celebs put on beach muscle for film roles all the time, only to lose it just as fast. But here was someone who was already a superstar busting it to become a real athlete, and completing 26.2 miles in four hours and 15 minutes with just eight weeks of preparation. And he lost five toenails!

So, yeah, the workout in this chapter is shorter than the others and has fewer moving parts, so to speak. It's nothing fancy, and that's exactly what's great about it. Basically, in addition to having you train your upper body one day a week and your lower body one day a week, I want you to hit it outdoors one day a week too.

How long, you ask? The duration of the outdoor session should be 45 minutes to an hour, just like the indoor workouts. The outdoor session is much more freestyle, though. You can do pretty much anything that elevates your heart rate significantly and fairly consistently for most of that time. Distance running is great, but so is interval training like wind sprints and hill runs. (Something like basketball isn't as good, because it's not constant—too much stop and go. Walking back to a starting line is one thing, but I don't want you standing there bent over, clutching your shorts with your hands.) For those of you living in the 'hood, don't get discouraged. I was living in the projects and I was still able to train outside. There's a park in every 'hood, and I've never seen a neighborhood that didn't have some stairs somewhere. No excuses—find a way!

Below, I'm going to provide some good options for accomplishing this, but keep in mind that you have an endless number of possibilities at your disposal, many of which are variations on running. Whether it was hills, stairs, intervals, or sprints, running was the most common form of cardiovascular training up through the 1960s. Later, people ditched it in favor of treadmills, stationary bikes, and step machines. My approach to training is old school in many respects, including this:

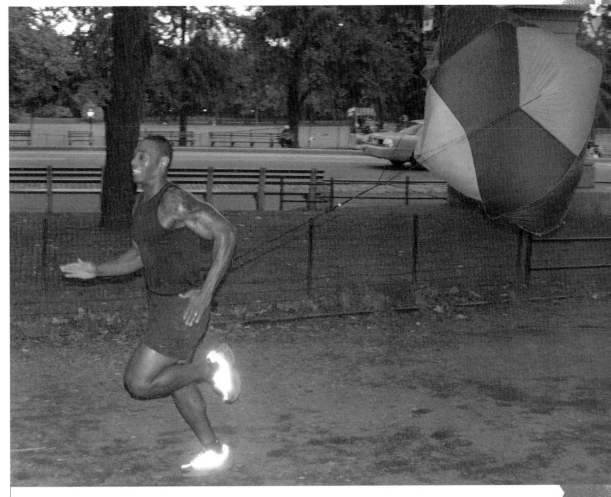

The parachute can create 100–200 pounds of drag while you sprint. It's not easy, but look at how much fun I'm having!

don't be afraid to go outside, put one foot in front of the other, and run some-times. Nothing against those machines—anything's better than nothing—but human beings have been running ever since they first ventured from caves to hunt, and it's worked pretty well ever since.

If you're new to outdoor training and haven't run outside since third grade phys-ed class, start slowly, because there's more to improving your running than

LIVE TO TRAIN ANOTHER DAY

It's a jungle out there, and for most of us, it's a concrete jungle. Here are some commonsense tips for surviving your training in the great outdoors.

Listen up. This one may be tough for some of you, but don't wear headphones when you're going to do roadwork of any kind, either on foot or on bicycle. If you're in a gym, feel free to listen to whatever you want. The same thing goes if you're running hills where cars aren't allowed. But when you're on the road, too many things can go wrong to be deaf to your surroundings. If a car's headed your way, you want to hear about it before it's too late. For the same reason, always run facing oncoming traffic. Safety first.

Buy good footwear. Don't skimp on quality when buying running shoes. Bad shoes can wreak all kinds of havoc on your training, not to mention on your feet. The more comfortable your feet are, the better you'll be able to perform. Also, applying Vaseline to your feet is a good way to prevent blisters. Take care of your feet. You need them 100 percent in these outdoor sessions, so you can really push it!

Don't isolate yourself in remote areas. You might be tempted to run off the beaten path sometimes, but don't go anywhere where no one will see you for minutes at a time. Remember, too, that darkness makes some places that are "public" during the day invisible at night. After dark, run or exercise in an area that's well lit.

Give someone a heads up. When possible, give someone a heads up when you leave for a jog. Tell them where you're going. Better yet, take a friend with you. If you can't find a human companion, your cell phone can be your best buddy.

When you go out to run, leave the ice in the jewelry box. Worry less about your appearance and more about not attracting muggers. It's a workout, not a fashion show.

Don't leave home without them—your cell phone and some ID, that is. The latter should include your name, phone number, and home address.

I know I've said it quite a few times already, but I can't stress it enough: **Safety first!**

just increasing your cardiovascular fitness. In the short term, your lungs may adapt more quickly than the rest of your body. That's why it's crucial that you let your joints and muscles adapt to the new stress they're going to be under.

The best way to do this is to build up your times slowly, even if your lungs can handle more stress. To begin, you don't want to run for as long as you can. Instead, you should begin with short, leisurely paced runs that allow your knees and other joints to grow accustomed to the demands you're placing on them. Take two to three weeks to settle in and get comfortable with your stride. By the third week, you should get a sense of how hard you can push and what your body can handle. Develop your instincts and listen to your body!

If you can't get through any of these outdoor workouts on the first go-round, that's cool. That's your motivation for next time. Let's say that while your ultimate goal is 45 minutes, the best you can manage initially is 10 minutes at a leisurely pace. (And we're not even assuming you can go that long.) The goal then becomes to increase your times gradually. You have to start somewhere. If you're still struggling with just that, take a buddy with you and motivate each other!

If you're trying to lose weight—particularly body fat—manipulate the pace and duration of your cardio sessions to maximize the benefit. It's true that lower-intensity cardio burns more fat as a *percentage* of total calories than higher-intensity cardio does, but the higher-intensity work burns more fat in the long run. That's because fast-paced running and interval sprinting burn more total calories, with a higher percentage coming from blood glucose. In contrast, walking burns a higher percent of calories from fat, but fewer calories total. So if you can only run for 20 minutes but will gladly walk for 40, walking is a better option for burning total fat calories. If you have only 20 minutes to exercise, do the activity that requires higher intensity. You can burn as much or more body fat, depending on how hard you push it. And I know you are going to push it!

Three final notes before moving onto the exercises: First, I encourage you to run on different surfaces. If you normally run on a track, try grass or sand instead. These can be more difficult because you get less spring on these softer surfaces, but they are easier on your joints.

Second, make sure you stretch after your outdoor sessions, or you may be too sore for the next one.

Third, have fun with it. This is not a boot-camp scenario. Make it pleasant, enjoy your surroundings, and breathe in that fresh air. But push yourself at the same time.

For each session, consider choosing one of the following (or make up your own drill):

1. UPHILL SPRINTS

Run up and walk down a hill 10 times. Make sure the walk-down is a measured pace. Don't stretch that out as you get tired. Time yourself. Try to run up the hill as fast as you can, then walk down to try to catch your breath. As soon as you hit the bottom again, it's on. Hustle right back up the hill. As well as being a potent fat burner, this builds and strengthens almost every muscle in your body, especially the glutes, thighs, and calves.

I beat up Mary with this one—there's a 50-yard hill right in front of her house.

2. PARACHUTE SPRINTS

One of my favorites. Run a series of sprints with a parachute trailing behind you, creating 100 to 200 pounds of drag, depending on which setting you use. If you're interested in purchasing a 'chute, visit performbetter.com. That's where I get mine.

Sprints without the parachute still work, but dragging it behind you is really challenging as well as fun. I use this one on my tough-guy clients.

3. INTERVALS

Running intervals can be as simple as walking the curves and running the straight parts of a track. Or you can interval-train by time, running for a minute, then walking for a minute. Another strategy for interval training is to adjust intensity, maybe going from a slow-paced run to a faster-paced run. Interval training is considered one of the most effective ways of burning fat. You can also do intervals on a bicycle. Do a 30-second sprint in a low gear, sprint for a minute in high gear to recover. Keep alternating between the two for the duration of your session. Intervals are great because they can be adapted to almost any type of cardiovascular machine on those bad-weather days.

EASY DOES IT!

If you've been training hard for any length of time, you already know your body doesn't respond to exercise as dramatically as it once did. Early on, you may have grown like a weed, but now that you've been at it for a minute, the gains are fewer and farther in between.

When your gains start to really diminish, or sometimes vanish, you might be suffering from what exercise specialists call *overtraining,* which is basically a breakdown in the recovery process. Any number of things can cause it; usually, it's some combination of excessive training, improper nutrition, insufficient sleep, and impaired recovery.

Here are some of the signs of overtraining.

❖ Elevated resting pulse rate in the morning
❖ Loss of interest in training
❖ Increased injuries, muscle aches, or both
❖ Irritability
❖ Insomnia
❖ Loss of muscle size
❖ Headaches
❖ Fatigue
❖ Diminished sex drive
❖ Loss of appetite
❖ Crankiness

Plenty of rest and attention to detail when it comes to nutrition are key for making sure this doesn't happen. Overtraining can turn you off to exercise because you're not getting results. It's important for anybody who's engaging in a workout program to get results regularly. It keeps your head in the game.

If you're not gaining, you might also be suffering from what is called *undertraining.* In layman's terms, this means you are slacking during your training sessions. But I know that you don't get down like that.

THE BUILDING BLOCKS

No split system works well indefinitely, so rearrange yours periodically. Here are some other aspects of the workout you can play with.

Exercise selection. Anyone who works out has literally hundreds of exercises from which to choose. However, they fall into two categories: Single-joint exercises, like the curl, require movement at only one joint or set or joints; multijoint exercises, like the squat, involve movement at more than one set of joints.

What this means to you: It's a good idea to master the basics (squats, curls, flyes, and the like) first, but over time, you'll need more tricks in your hat. Read more fitness books and magazines. Continue your fitness education. It's your body. Knowledge is power!

Volume. Although poundage is often included in a technical definition of volume, basically it's the sum total of the sets times the reps for each exercise you do in any workout.

What this means to you: You can manipulate volume by increasing or decreasing reps, sets or both.

Repetitions. You complete one rep when you move a load (even if it's just your body) from a starting position through the movement itself and then back to the starting position. If you take that movement to the point of full contraction and back, you've gone through what's called full range of motion. Anything less amounts to a partial rep.

Regardless, each rep has a concentric half, during which the working muscle shortens. (In the case of a dumbbell curl, you flex your elbow to raise the weight.) It also has an eccentric half, during which the working muscle lengthens. (For the same exercise, you extend your elbow joint to lower the weight back down.) If you go for what's called a peak contraction in between those halves, you're generating an isometric contraction at the midpoint of the rep.

What this means to you: Higher reps—say, more than 15 per set—are good for building muscle endurance. For making muscles bigger, sets in the range of 8 to 15 work best. Sets of fewer than eight reps will emphasize the development of pure strength. Power lifters, in fact, will do one- or two-rep sets.

Sets. The reps you do consecutively before stopping constitute one set.

What this means to you: You don't want to do dozens of sets, like Arnold did in his heyday, but you want to do a few sets for each exercise to make sure you really hit the muscle.

Frequency. This refers to intervals at which you train different parts of your body. If you train abs three times a week, for example, you train them frequently. If you train them three times a month, you train them less frequently.

What this means to you: Never train a muscle when it's still sore from a prior workout. Beginners probably shouldn't train more than three times a week, and even intermediates probably shouldn't exceed four weekly sessions. Experienced lifters with an informed approach to nutrition and recuperation often can avoid overtraining even when working out with great frequency by just listening to their body.

Intensity. Intensity is a catchall that encompasses any variable that can make your workout more or less difficult, including volume, weight, between-sets rest, and tempo.

What this means to you: Your goal should be to increase the amount of weight you lift gradually over time. If you're a guy and you want to get bigger, that's really the only way you're going to do it. For women, you may want to decrease rest times in between sets while increasing your repetitions. High intensity doesn't always mean heavy weight!

Train hard but train smart. Stick to the program, and eliminate the guesswork! This is $1500-an-hour information!

4. STAIRS

If your gym has a StepMill, then you may already know how challenging *walking* stairs can be. On the average stair stepper, you aren't required to lift your entire bodyweight. The stair stepper sinks slowly, assisting you against gravity. Out in the real world, no such luck.

Find the longest set of stairs you can find, whether that's along or inside a building, or at a nearby stadium. Start out walking from the bottom to the top, and then come back down. You'll notice a large change in your heart rate between the ascent and descent. This is ideal interval training as well.

Allow yourself to get comfortable walking the stairs before you attempt to run them. When you get in better shape, run up and slowly walk back down.

GETTING UNSTUCK

If you're not making gains, do not quit. Each of the following strategies can help you get rolling again.

- ❖ If you've been killing yourself in the gym to no avail, forget about training for a week. Focus your mind on other pressing matters instead, like solving world hunger or figuring out why TV detectives can only solve crimes once they've been kicked off the force.
- ❖ If, on the other hand, too many days off every week is the problem, blast your body for a week or so. Let it know you're back in charge.
- ❖ Get adequate sleep, which means *at least* eight hours a night.
- ❖ Eat five or six healthy, nutrient-packed meals a day. You're not going anywhere if you don't have fuel in your tank.
- ❖ Give your body adequate time to rest in between workouts. Seldom, if ever, train the same body part on back-to-back days, for example.

5. SPRINTS

You can start off sprinting for 100 to 200 yards, and then walk for a minute or two in between. As your body adapts to this training regimen, decrease your rest periods. Try to imagine yourself running away from your old body and chasing down the new you. This really motivates me to run faster!

6. AGILITY DRILLS

These can be as simple as taking a ball, throwing it against the wall, and then chasing it down and catching it. You can do a set of 30 reps, rest, and then hit it again. Or take some chalk and outline a ladder in the street, and run through it. Shadowbox! Park benches are often in a row, and you can slide side to side among them in lateral motion. Or you can hop up on a bench and step back down.

Try doing, say, 10 minutes of each one of these, until you reach your target of 45 minutes to an hour.

It's all about getting your heart rate up, improving your agility, and getting some fresh air.

7. JUMPING ROPE

Everyone has probably jumped rope at some point in his or her life, but not everyone has done it correctly. The most important thing is to choose a rope that's long enough. Put your foot down on the middle of the rope, and then pull the ends up toward you. If the rope is long enough, the ends will reach up to your chest. Once you begin jumping, keep your elbows in toward your sides. Remember, you only have to jump as high as the rope is thick.

Not only does this burn fat, it improves your timing, builds your shoulders, and increases your speed. You can also develop signature moves and cool tricks.

If you think this is only for little girls, you're wrong. Just go to any boxing gym and see what they use for conditioning. This is also one that Mr. Combs and I used in our preparation for the marathon. Five minutes equals 1 mile, with minimum impact. You can't beat that!

How to Get LL Cool J's Total Package

The same drive that has sustained LL's musical life for 19 years—an eternity in hip-hop—has also allowed him to build the best body in the industry. Sure, he cranks up his training and dieting periodically for a film role or a concert tour, but he trains and eats correctly year-round. LL is different from the others. He could have been a pro body-builder, a boxer, or an NFL linebacker if he had set his mind to any of those goals. LL Cool J is an athlete who happens to make his living as an entertainer.

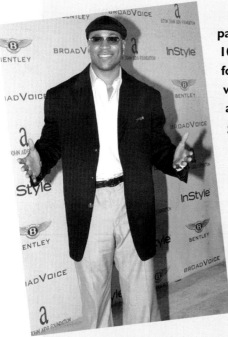

His secret to achieving the total package you see in films and on videos is 100 percent dedication, which takes the form of strict dieting and balls-to-the-wall training! It also manifests itself in an incredible attention to detail. He gets his eight hours of rest a night, always takes his vitamins—and does all that sort of unglamorous-but-critical stuff. He's incredibly strong mentally and spiritually, too. His faith in God and his belief in himself fuel him even when he's running on E. All of the above permeates everything he does, and that's why he has the total package.

You already have the program you need for achieving the same. In fact, you're holding it in your hands. But don't hesitate to add a few twists from LL's bag of tricks. For example, try doing some box-ing. To go 15 rounds, boxers treat aerobic and anaerobic as two sides of the same coin, just like I do in *The Jump Off*. LL is a fighter at heart, and he trains like one, too.

Include a boxing circuit in your regimen each week. Sequence, for example, four minutes of shadowboxing; a minute of push-ups; a minute of sit-ups, where you're catching a medicine ball at the top; and then two minutes of jumps and bounds wearing a weighted vest. LL does five or six such circuits in one session. Build up your strength and endurance to where you're repeating the cycle.

Also, do some interval training. If you don't know it by now, you can stoke the fat-burning furnace with intervals, which simply involve varying your aerobic workout intensity systematically (not randomly). Instead of doing your cardio steady state this week, do it for two minutes with your heart rate above 150 beats per minute, followed by one minute at 135 to 140, and so on, until you run out of steam. If you're not doing it already, start measuring your heart rate during cardio.

And no matter what, keep doin' it and doin' it—even when you don't feel like doin' it. This is the most important lesson you can learn from LL Cool J. The key to getting in shape is eating right when you don't feel like it and working out when you don't feel like it. Feel me?

So what are you waiting for? Get yours!

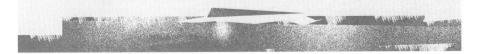

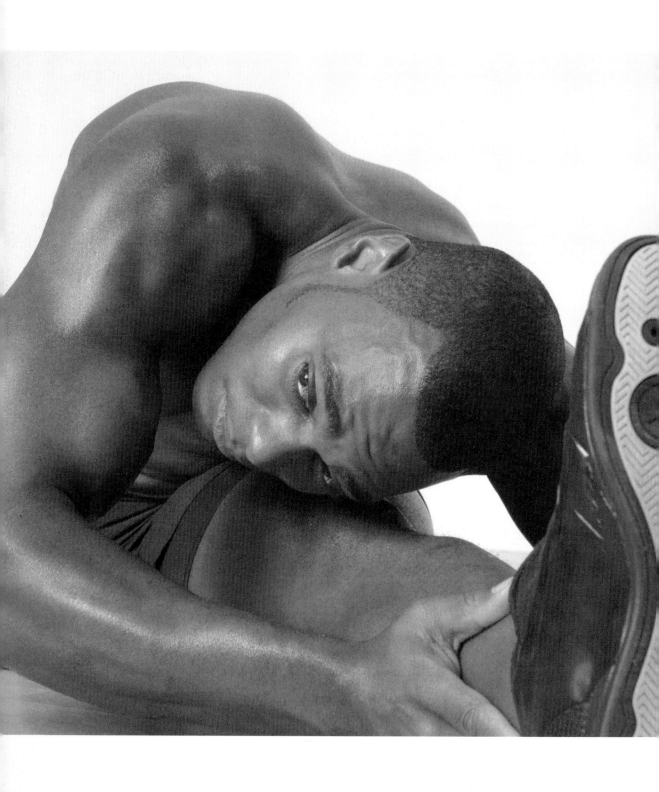

Flexibility Training—Bent into Shape

You've pumped iron hard and hit the intervals hard, so don't spoil it by neglecting to stretch. Flexibility training is just as important as the weights and cardio, so put 100 percent into it. A healthy muscle is a flexible muscle. You need to stretch after every workout. So don't blow by this chapter. Read it!

Stretching is the act of lengthening your muscles and connective tissues, particularly the tendons and ligaments. Stretch a muscle far enough and a reflex automatically makes it tighten up, but repetition gradually allows you to improve your range of motion. Connective tissues in particular become more brittle as you get older, particularly after 40. Formerly problem-free joints and muscles can get a little rusty and stiff without use. This is your body telling you to start stretching, and if you don't, you're setting yourself up for injury and bad posture—not a good look!

The benefits of stretching are many. First and foremost is injury prevention. Having more flexibility will improve your performance, whether you're shooting a jumper, throwing a kick, driving a golf ball, or having sex. Some intriguing research also suggests that people who stretch after lifting weights gain more strength than those who don't.

There are many different kinds of stretching methods available. *Static* stretches are the most basic. Picture the traditional toe touch, where you stretch to the farthest point possible and then hold that position for 10 to 30 seconds. Then there are *ballistic* stretches, where you reach out to touch your toes and then try to increase the range of motion by bouncing back and forth. *Dynamic* stretches typically involve gentler, more sports-specific motions such as a swimmer taking his shoulder through a swirling motion or a sprinter mimicking a high knee kick. If you start off an exercise in the gym with a set using little or no weight—maybe just the bar—you're really performing a dynamic stretch, if you think about it. Then there are some really fancy forms of assisted stretching with names like *active-isolated* and *proprioceptive neuromuscular facilitation (PNF)*, all of which require the services of a training partner. I'm not going to ask you to do something I can barely pronounce, so we're going to implement the KISS system of stretching: Keep It Simple, Stupid.

Different stretching styles are suited for particular sports or forms of exercise. Static stretches can help any athlete and may be sufficient by themselves for simple, repetitive activities like jogging and cycling. Dynamic stretching is well suited for warming up a complicated joint like the shoulder for sports such as swimming and volleyball. Active-isolated and PNF are great for the pros, who go though extreme and sometimes awkward ranges of motion in games. For the Jump Off, we're going to go with the old-school basics, relying on a combination of static and dynamic stretches. Avoid ballistic stretches, where you're bouncing. That's how you pull a muscle. All you need to do is be flexible enough not to injure yourself and survive these hard-core sessions.

Stretch for a good 15 minutes or more at the end of every workout, whether it's upper body, lower body, or the outdoors session. Better yet, do another five minutes of stretching even on days when you don't train. Many office workers sit hunched in front of a computer five days a week, and it's terrible for their posture. Believe me, only five minutes a day can help.

I'm asking you to stretch at the end of the workouts, rather than the beginning. I prefer the end because by that time your blood flow and body temperature have increased. Before the workout, stretching a cold muscle, you're more likely to injure yourself. After the workout, when your muscles and connective tissues are at their most elastic, you can really increase your range of motion, as well as hasten recovery and lessen muscle soreness.

Do the following stretches in order after the last set of your workout, with no rest in between, and you'll be good to go. Don't be afraid to improvise, though. If your quads are tight, do more quad stretches. If your hamstrings are tight, do more hamstring stretches. Get it? All stretches are done on the floor except as noted.

1. SUNRISE SPINE STRETCH

This is a yoga-inspired stretch. Place your palms and knees on the ground so that your arms and thighs are parallel with each other and your torso is parallel with the ground. Inhale as you draw your torso up, causing your spine to arch slightly, like a frightened cat. Exhale and raise your head up as you push your torso down, at which point your stomach will be trying to hit the ground. **Inhale on the way up, exhale on the way down, and repeat three times.**

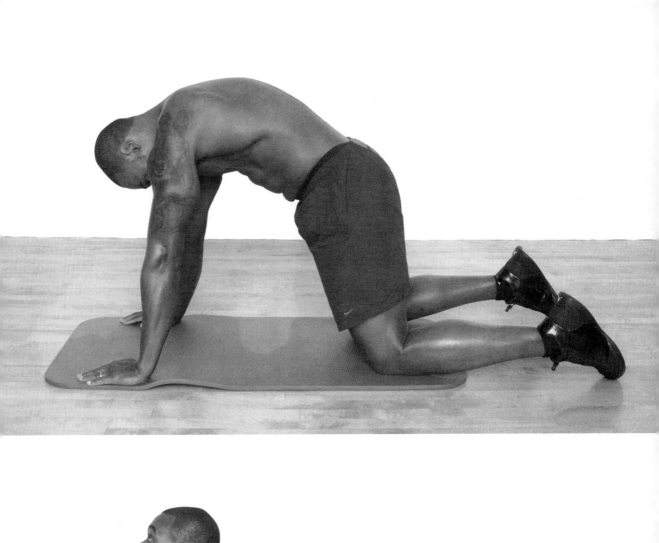

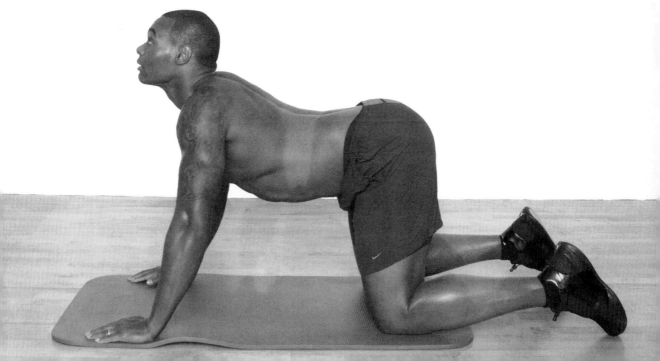

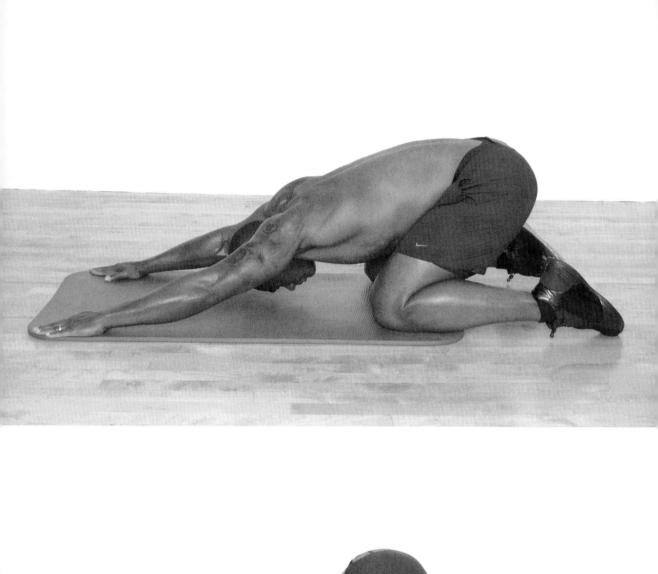

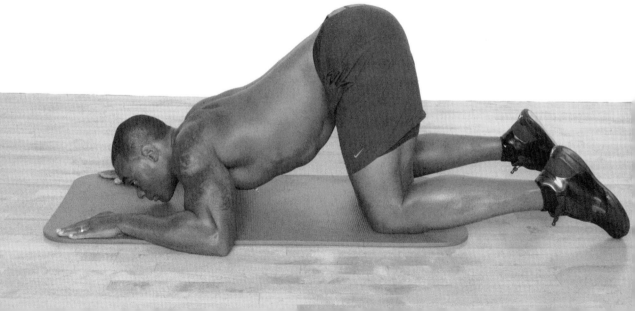

Start in the same position as the spinal stretch, but then sit back and lower your torso to the floor, face-down, with your arms extended in front of you. Your chest should be touching the tops of your thighs, and your back should be rounded slightly. Keeping your palms in the same position and your chest as close to the floor as possible, arch all the way through, raising your torso at the end like a cobra. Rotate your torso gently from side to side to stretch your abs as well. Exhale as you go through the stretch.

Do it three times, breathing slower and more deeply each time.

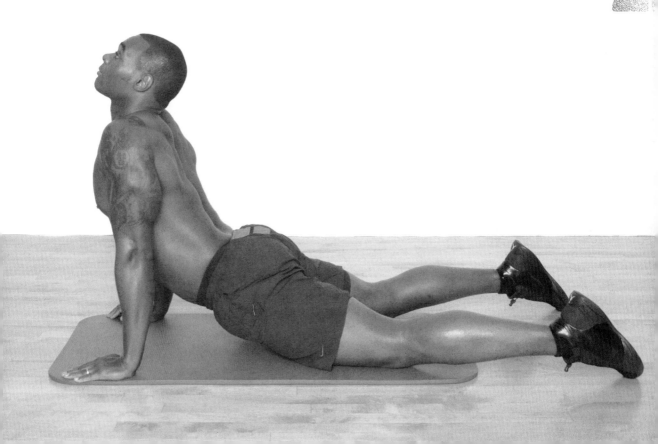

3. QUAD STRETCH

As soon as you finish those, lie face-down on the floor. Reach back with one hand and grab the ankle of that leg. Extend the other arm in front of you. Feel the muscle in your leg stretch; connect your mind to it. Hold it for a 10 count and then repeat using the other hand and leg.

Three sets, 10 seconds each leg. Breathe and feel the tension leave your body!

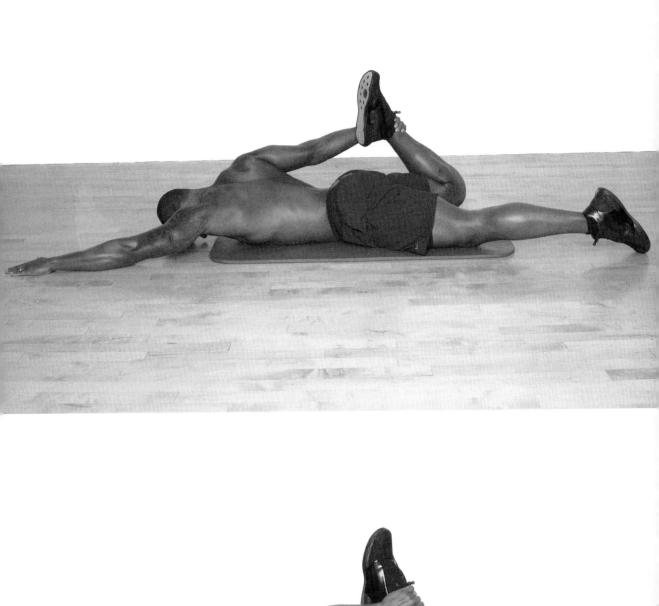
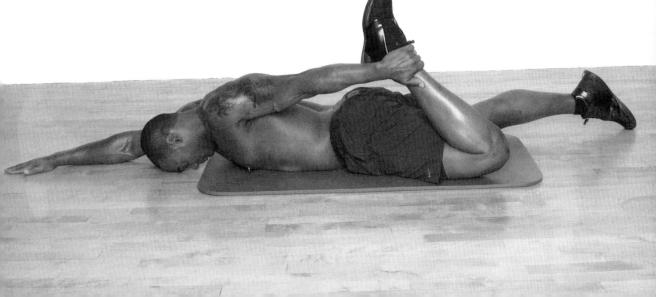

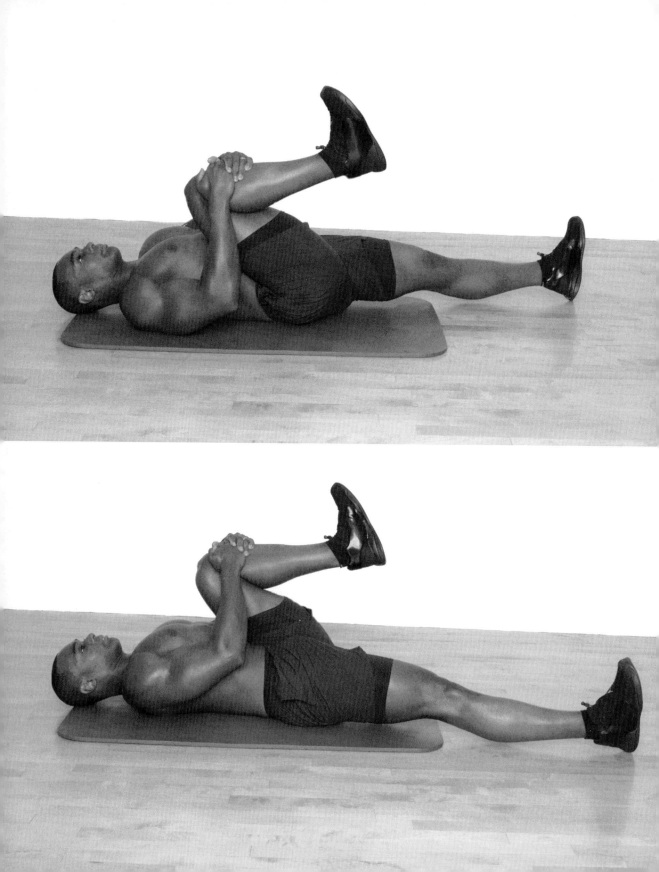

4. HAMSTRING STRETCH

Roll over onto your back, so that your legs are extended. Raise one leg until you can grasp that knee with both hands. (Be sure to keep the opposing leg on the floor, so you get a full stretch.) Keeping your head and shoulders on the floor, pull the knee into the chest, hold for a 10 count, and then release. Repeat using the other leg.

Fill and empty those lungs!

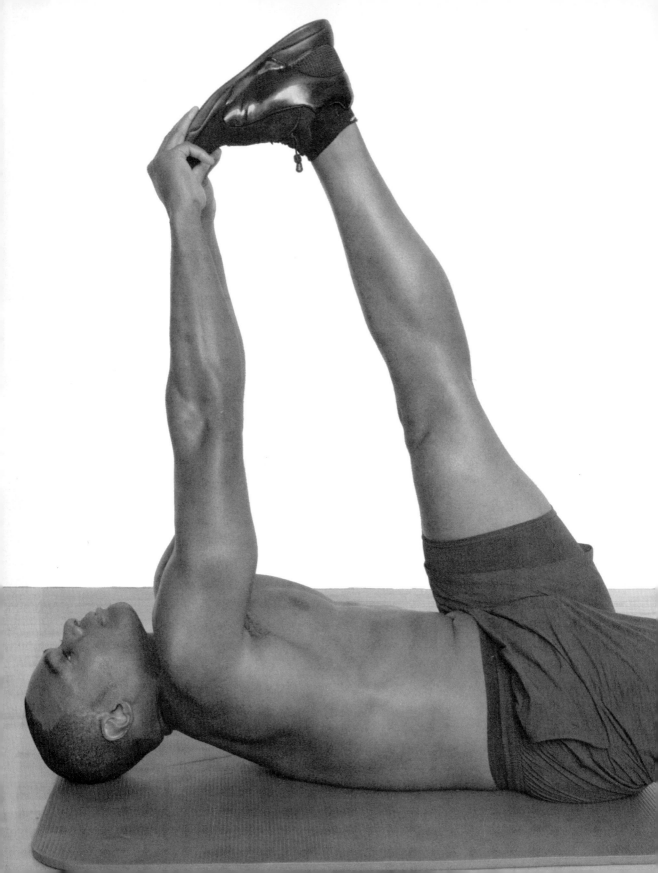

Use the same position as above, only keep your working leg straight—don't bend it. With both hands now grasp your toes, not your knee. Pull the toe gently toward your head, which stretches the calf as well. Try to keep your back flat. Same goes for the leg not being stretched. **Use a towel if you can't reach your toes.**

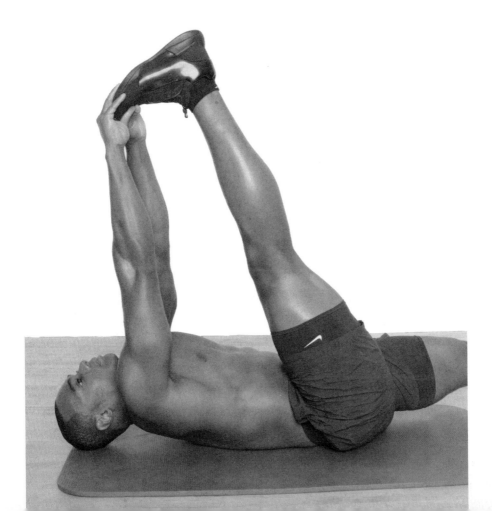

6. INNER-THIGH STRETCH

Remain flat on your back, but raise both knees up toward you, grasping each one with a hand. Gently pull your legs out to the sides, feeling the stretch in your inner thigh muscles. Hold it for a 10 count. **Think about what a winner you are for training!**

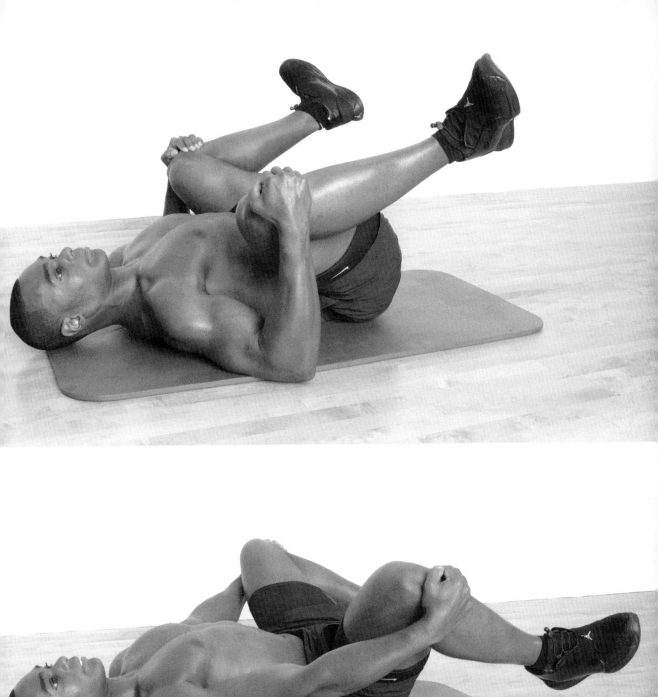
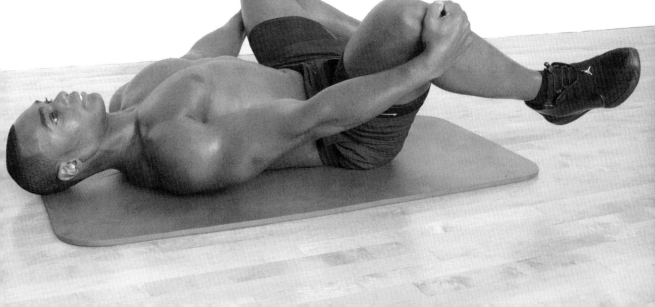

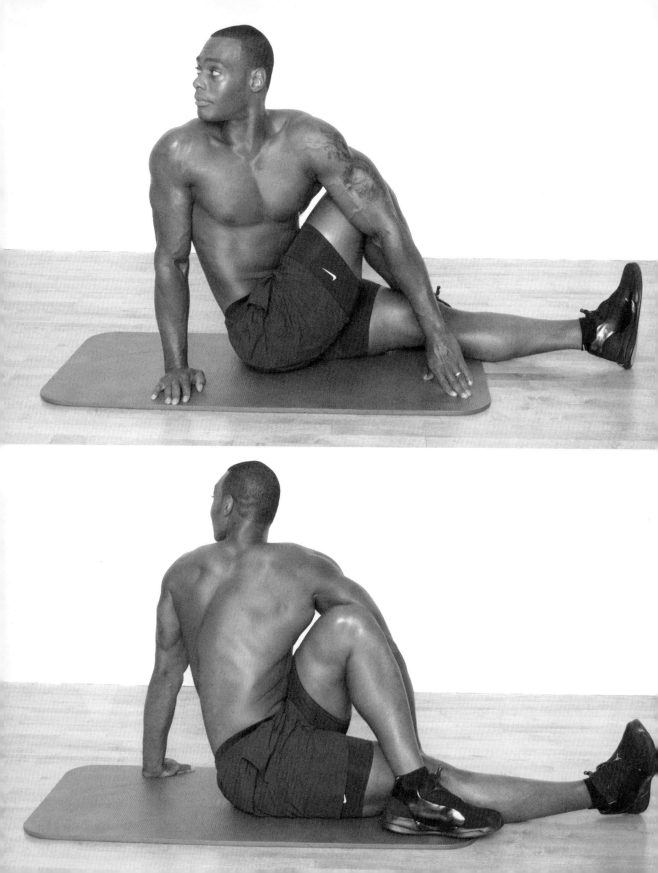

7. BACK STRETCH

Sit up so that your torso is upright and your legs are extended out in front of you. Pull your right leg across your left so that your right heel is right next to your left knee, and then rotate your torso to the right, so your left elbow is up against your right knee. Hold for 10 seconds. **Reverse the position and hold for another 10 seconds. Have a sip of water between stretches.**

8. LOWER-BACK AND HIP STRETCH

From the same starting position as the back stretch above, lean forward, wrap your fingers over your toes, and hold for 10 seconds. **No bouncing! Slow and controlled.**

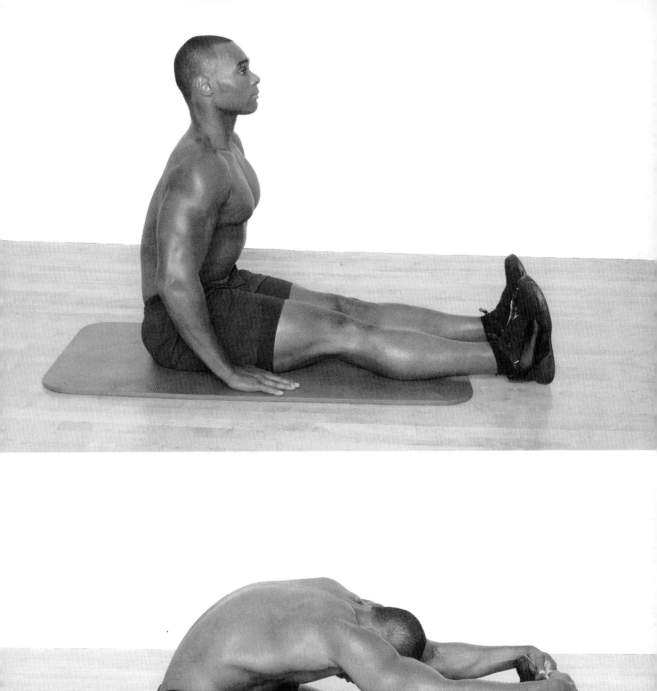

9. GROIN STRADDLE STRETCH

Slowly sit up, extending your legs out into a V. Slowly reach toward one foot with both hands. Hold momentarily. Slowly reach toward the other foot with both hands. Slowly reach to the center with both hands. Repeat this progression several times. **Go deeper in the stretch with each repetition.**

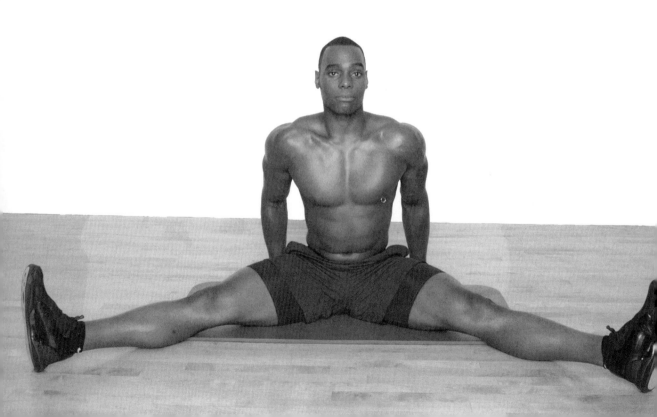

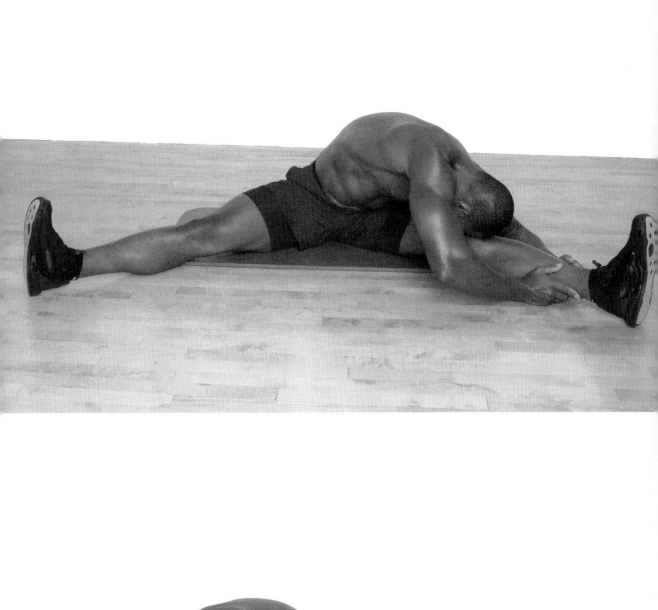

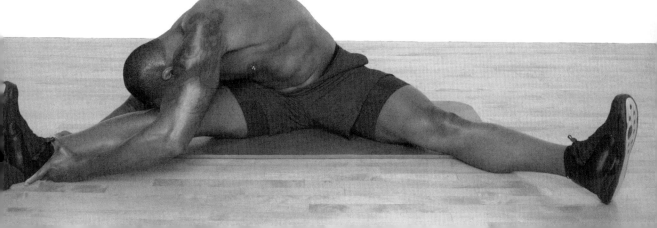

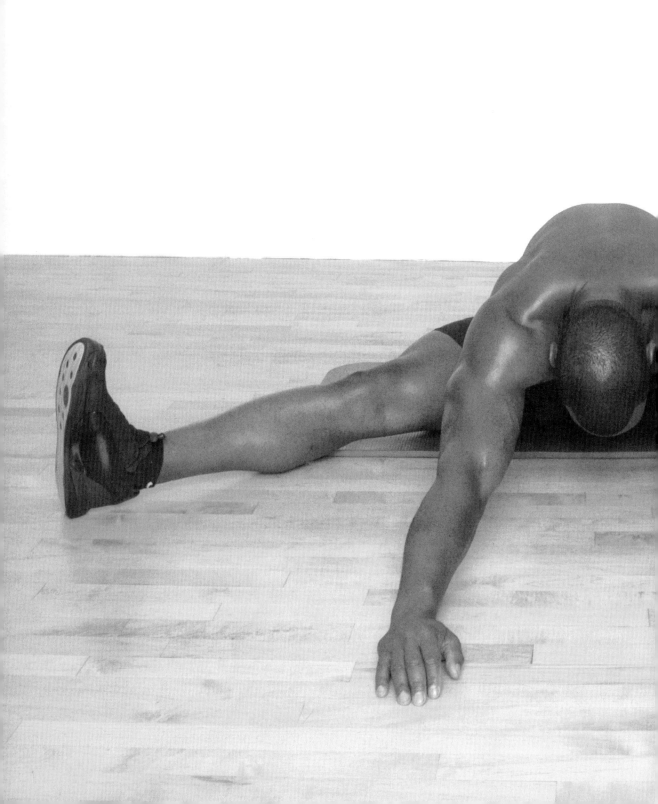

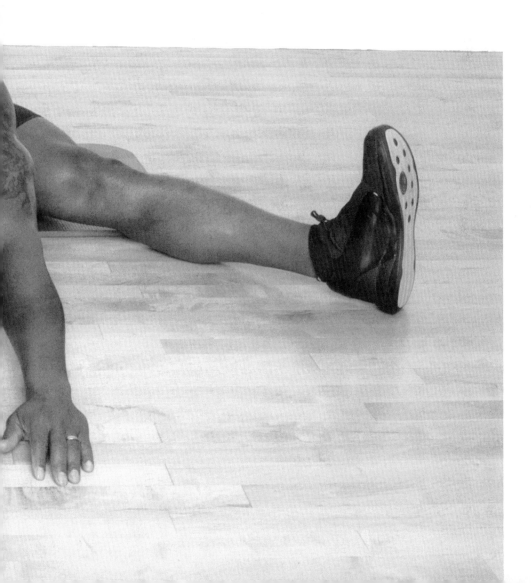

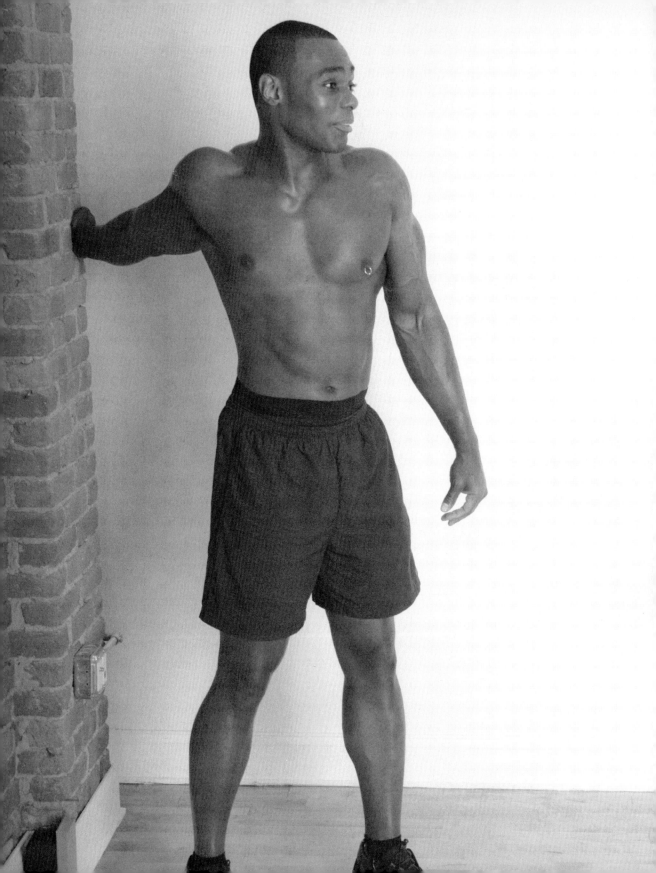

10. CHEST STRETCH

Standing with your feet shoulder-width apart, reach over and grasp a wall or support with one hand, with the other arm hanging at your side. The extended arm should be slightly behind the plane of your torso. Slowly rotate your torso a few inches away from the support and hold. Repeat using the opposite arm. **Visualize your new hard body.**

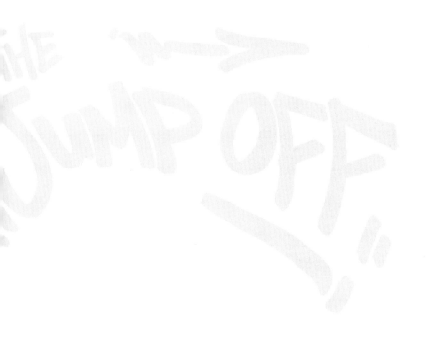

11. SHOULDER STRETCH

From that same starting position, extend one of your arms out in front of you. Take your other arm, and, keeping the elbow of the extended arm fixed, pull that arm toward you, gently. Hold it for a few seconds and then return to the starting position. **Repeat using the opposite arm.**

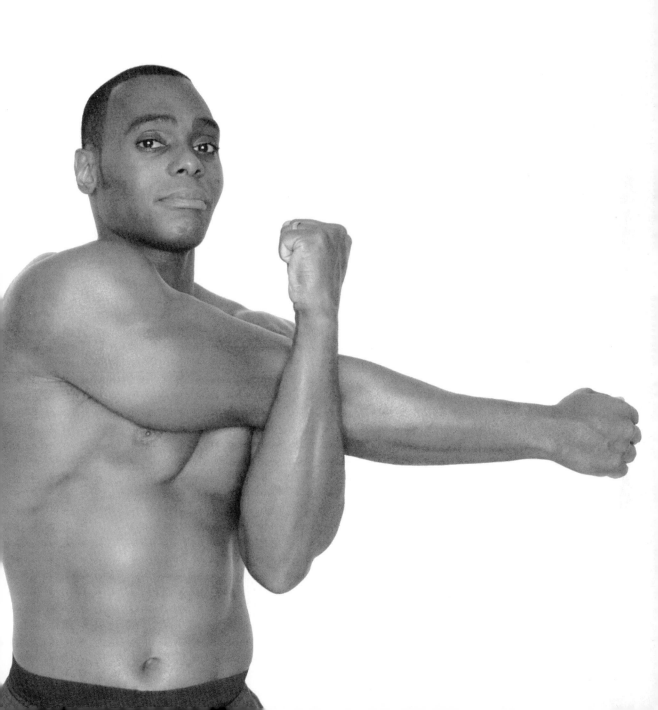

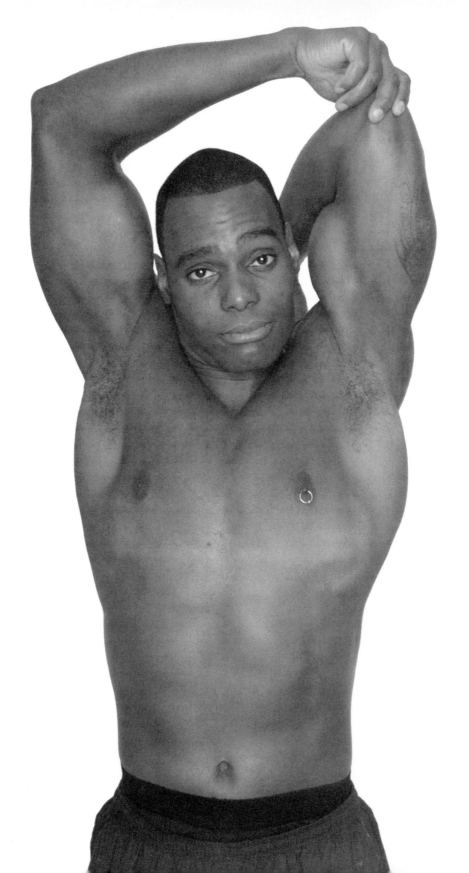

12. TRICEPS STRETCH

Lift one arm and bend your elbow so that your hand comes back behind your head. Grab that triceps with your other arm and gently push it back as far as it can comfortably go. Hold for the time it takes you to inhale deeply two or three times. Reverse arm positions and repeat. **Use a towel if this is too difficult.**

13. STANDING SPINE STRETCH

Stand with your feet slightly wider than shoulder-width apart, toes angled out ever so slightly. Your arms should be at your sides. Bend at the knees to descend into a squat, basically, but as your thighs approach parallel, round your back and lower your head so that it ends up between your calves and you're staring at the ground. Slowly return to the starting position and repeat. **Focus on fluid motion and deep breathing.**

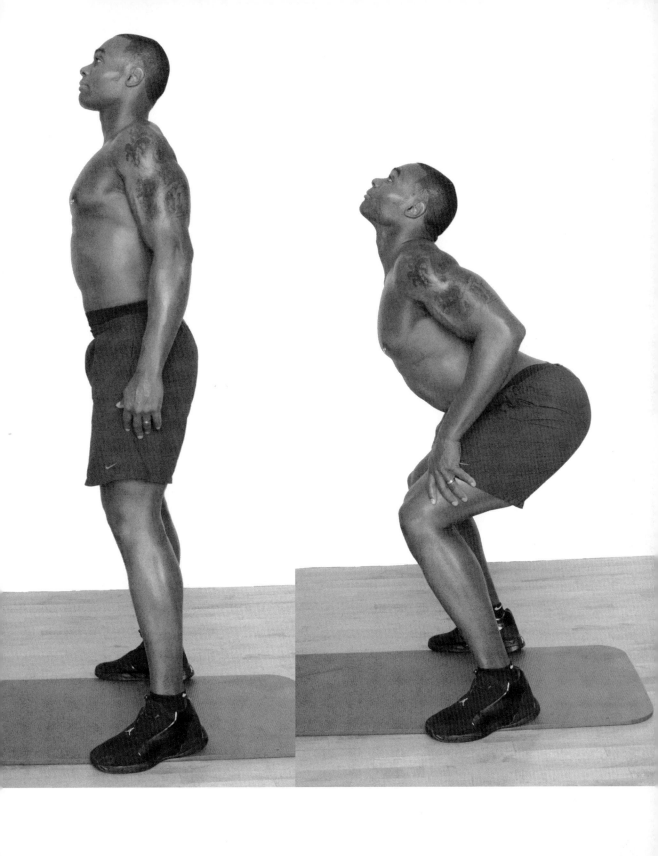

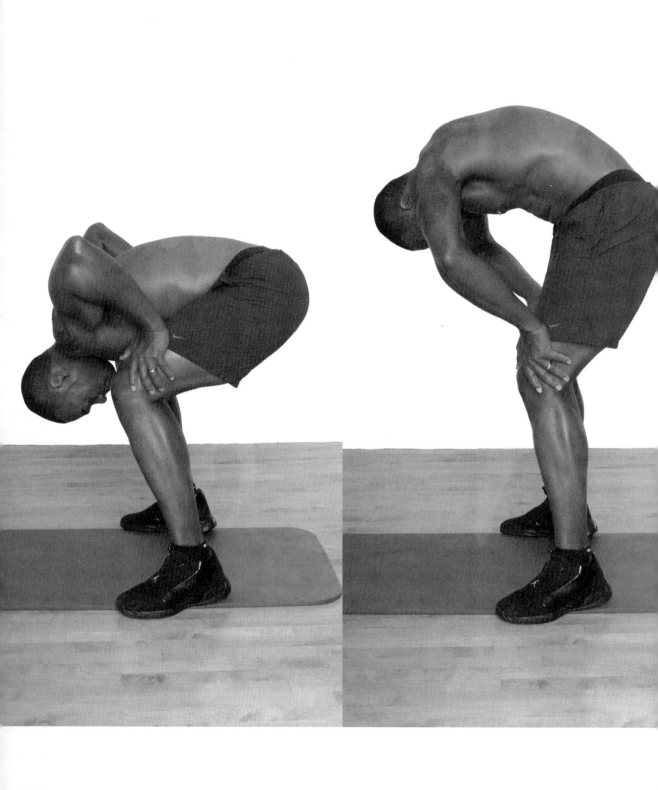

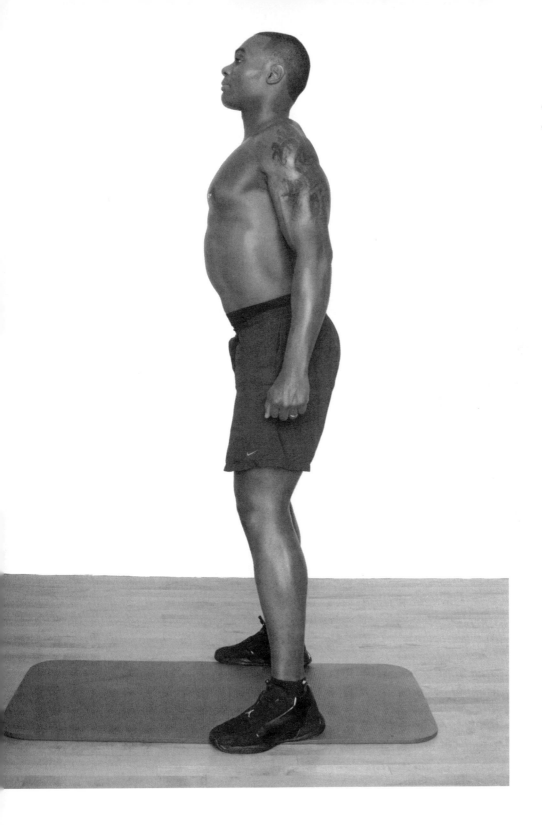

14.
NECK STRETCH

Stay in the same position, but this time, rotate your neck four or five times. **Stop and do the same number of rotations in the direction counter to what you just did.**

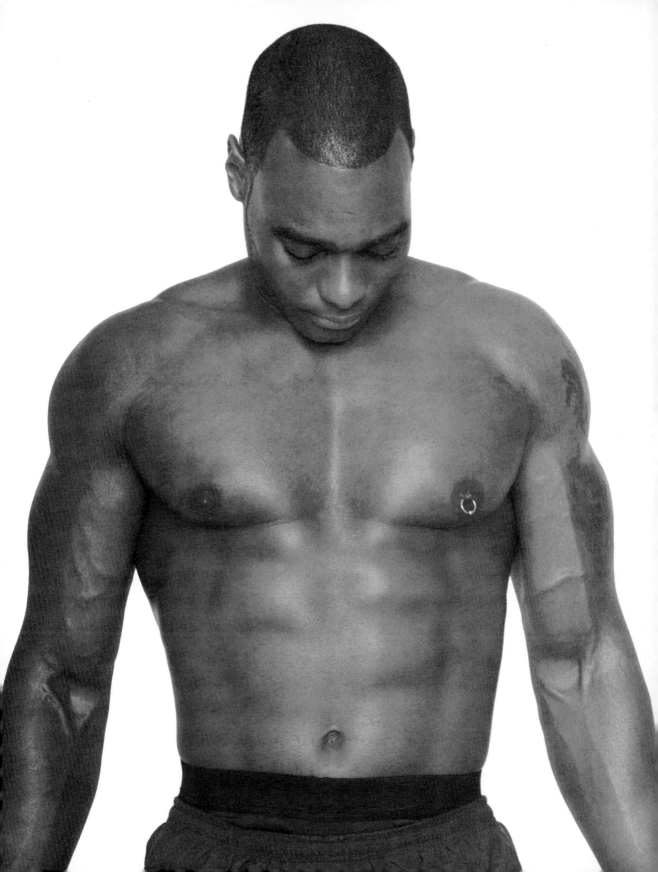

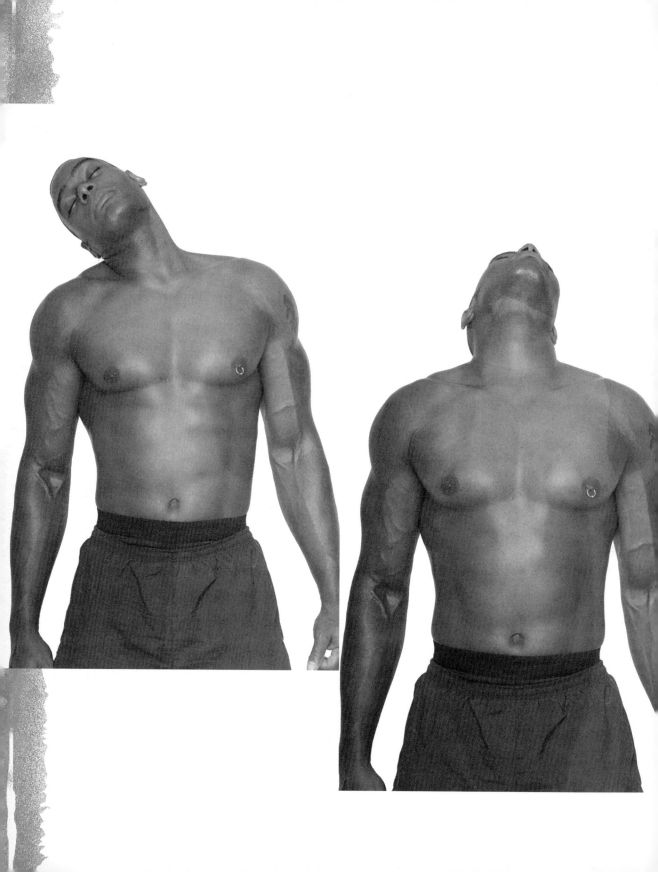

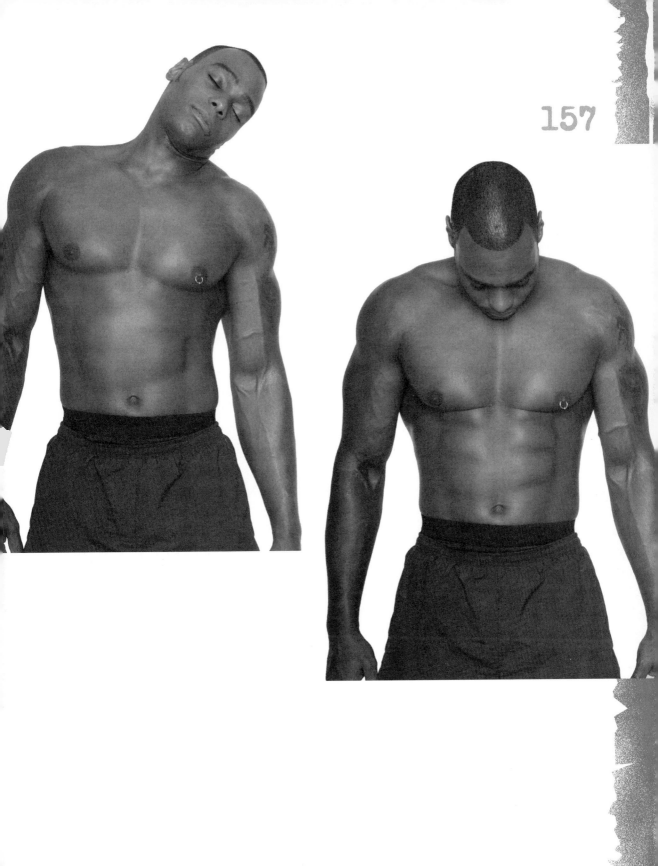

15.

CONGRATULATORY STRETCH

Assume the same position as the triceps stretch, but this time pat yourself on the back with the hand trailing behind your head (not pictured).

Good workout, guys. Follow up with proper diet and that hard body is yours!

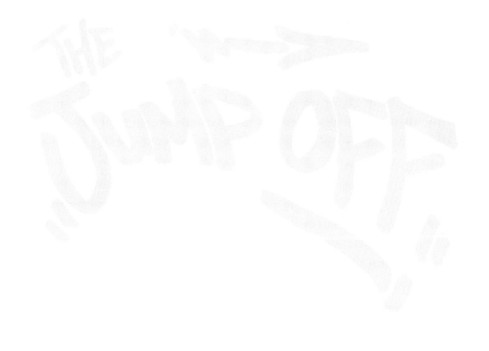

JOINT VENTURES

Compound movements are what exercise physiologists call movements that occur at more than one joint or set of joints in your body. That may sound complicated, but it's really very simple. Here's the deal: When you squat or lunge, for example, your hips, knees, and ankles all flex as you descend and then extend to bring your body back up. Because they help develop coordination and typically allow you to use heavier weights, compound movements generally do a better job of developing muscle size, strength, and coordination than single-joint exercises do. That's why compound movements predominate in the lower-body workout I've designed for you.

Single-joint exercises, as the name suggests, involve movement across only one joint or set of joints. Picture a calf raise. If performed using strict form, only your ankle joints should move. With a few notable exceptions—for example, an Olympic weight lifter training for a competition—a well-balanced, complete resistance training program should include at least some single-joint movements. They allow you to zero in on and tire out individual muscles and muscle groups in a way that multijoint exercises often cannot. On the multijoint squat, for example, your quads will often fail before your glutes. Following up that exercise with the single-joint one like the glute squeeze will further target, and exhaust, that booty!

No Pain, No Gain?
Think Again!

Train hard, but stop short of injuring yourself.
That advice might sound obvious to the point of insulting your intelligence, but remember that an injury can manifest itself not only in acute pain but also in soreness from tissue damage that materializes in the days following a workout. If you overextend yourself early on, you'll know it when you can't get out of bed the next day.

The question facing beginners is how to distinguish between acceptable and unacceptable levels of pain. As you train a body part, the "burn" you feel in a muscle reflects a build-up of lactic acid. That's acceptable. As a general rule, when you start to feel discomfort in the joints instead of in the muscle, it's usually time to put the weight down.

The generalized soreness you feel after workout, which is normal, is called delayed onset muscle soreness (DOMS). It reflects trauma experienced by muscles you just worked. The challenge is differentiating DOMS, which is uncomfortable but doesn't inflict any permanent damage, from more serious problems, such as tendonitis (inflammation of a tendon) or muscle strain. Duration is the key. DOMS typically becomes noticeable 24 hours after a workout, peaks at around 48 hours, and should be dissipating 72 hours out from a training session. If the pain is getting worse rather than improving after three days, and/or you reach a point where the limb or body part isn't functional for routine tasks, you should definitely seek medical help.

By the time most people seek medical help, they're beyond DOMS and into the realm of more debilitating injuries. Usually it's some kind of overuse or overtraining injury like tendonitis or tenosynovitis, an inflammation of a tendon. Treatment can range from rest and the application of heat or cold to immobilization of the affected area.

By just paying attention to your body and following the guidelines in *The Jump Off,* you can avoid injury and unnecessary discomfort.

How to Get Endurance Like P. Diddy

The secret to P. Diddy's endurance lies in his ability to commit completely to any challenge or project he takes on. Mentally, the man is a monster!

When we first hooked up, Puffy was somewhat overweight, and his knees couldn't really take a major pounding. So I started him doing 15 minutes of intervals on the stationary bike, where he'd alternate 30 seconds of cruising with 30 seconds of sprinting done at the highest resistance. By that final 30-second blast, his heart would be pumping at 175 beats per minute! Puff's body adapted quickly, so I increased the intensity by adding a minute to the duration every two sessions, and by switching him over to a more demanding machine every few weeks.

Then one day we were talking about training, and I told him that every true Renaissance man has either run a marathon or run with the bulls in Spain. I suggested he consider doing the New York City Marathon, and I told him it would be cool to do it for charity! Now, I suggest this to every client I train, but in 10 years, he's the only one who has taken me up on it. The next day, he had everything arranged! Eight weeks later we would run it, and the rest is history.

We started off by doing 1 1/2 miles around the Central Park Reservoir. Then we went around it twice, doubling the distance to 3 miles.

One day, I was like, "Man, let's run the whole park."

He was like, "Are you *crazy?*"

The whole park was 6.2 miles, so we made that jump next, and then just kept building it up from there.

Bring Puffy's hunger out in yourself and you can run a marathon with only eight weeks of training, just like we did! To get there, you only need to do a long run once a week, along with a series of shorter, more intense runs. In fact, I advise against running distance more than once a week, because running is very psychological, and you don't want to turn it into drudgery. What you can do is add to your cardiovascular efficiency by jumping rope indoors in between runs. That way, each run, you'll be able to see improvement in your conditioning and go a little farther. So you end up seeing progress from the beginning of the week to the end of the week, with some indoor cardio in the middle giving you a nice change of pace along the way.

One final note: If you're out running and you run out of gas, it's okay to walk for a while instead, but don't start draggin' ass— keep your arms pumping! Power walk. You *have* to keep your heart rate up somehow. No excuses! Once you catch your breath, pick it up again. Don't quit!

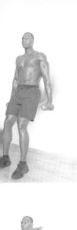

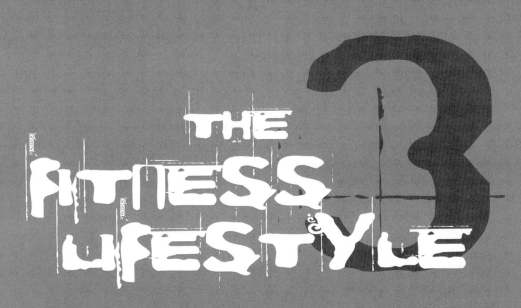

THE FITNESS LIFESTYLE

3

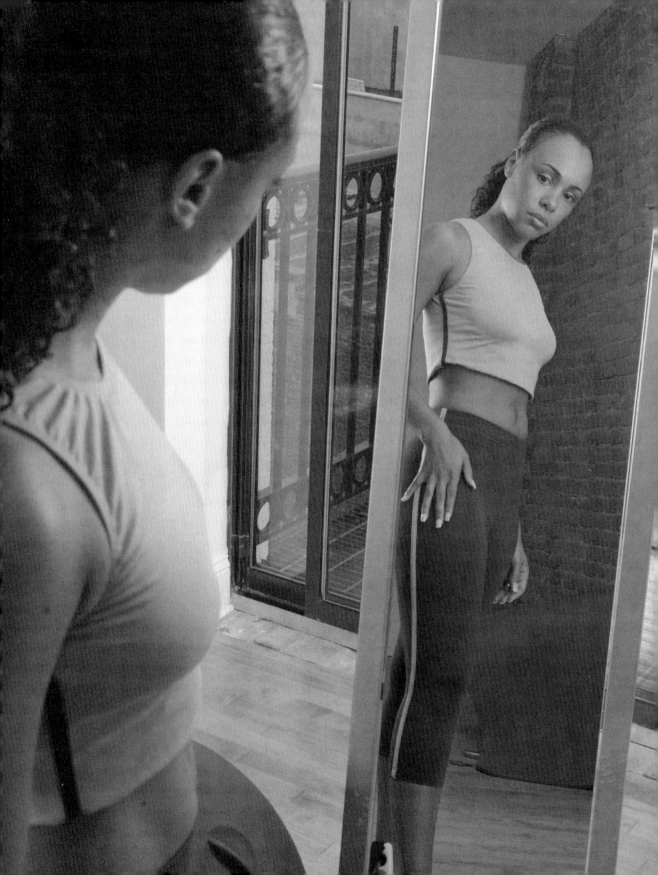

Nutrition— You Really Are What You Eat

Eat carbs.

Don't eat carbs.

Never eat fat.

Eat according to your blood type.

Eat 8 ounces of lean, organic barbecue ribs on a paper plate by the light of a full moon, naked.

Okay, that last one I made up, but with all these insane theories about diet and nutrition flying around, it's harder than ever to find a grain of truth buried under all the BS. But marketing hype and fad diets aside, the fact remains that 80 percent of your success with any fitness program is anchored in your diet. Straight up: You can train 'til the cows come home, but you'll still look like a load if you're eating buckets of KFC. To get the most out of your training, you need to stoke your metabolism with the proper fuel.

But diet and nutrition aren't only about looking good and fitting into those jeans and throwbacks. It's about living your life to its fullest, longest, healthiest potential. Every year, a ridiculously high percentage of the African American population dies as a direct result of poor nutritional habits. That Southern cooking may taste amazing, but eventually it'll kill you. *Everything* is fried. They'll fry an apple if given half a chance. And the West Indian diet is just as bad. It's no wonder diabetes, cardiovascular disease, and stroke claim the lives of thousands of us each year, every year. The sad thing is, many of those deaths could have been prevented with some simple dietary changes.

So whether you want to look good, feel good, live longer, or all of the above, formulating a solid nutritional plan is the way to go. But before we get into that, let me give you some added motivation.

Feed Your Mind

If you've ever seen anyone on one of those low-carb or carb-free diets, you've probably noticed that they're distracted, spacey, even moody, to the point where you'll go out of your way to avoid them. They're not forgetting to take their Prozac—they're just suffering from brain drain. Literally. Your brain runs exclusively on glucose, and if you're on a low-carb or carb-restrictive diet, your blood sugar will inevitably fall below comfortable levels. When you're in this hypoglycemic state, your brain will begin to complain. You'll feel dizzy, crabby, irritable, shaky, nervous, hungry, nauseated, even depressed until you get the sugar fix you need. So force-feed those carb-free fools a baked potato and see how quickly they lose their 'tude! And you'll still get your hard body!

SCARY STATS

I put these down to shake you up a bit. If they scare you into taking action, they're having the desired effect. The health issues facing the African American community require that we focus special attention on our diet. Remember, there's a direct correlation between your eating, how long you live, and the quality of your life.

In the United States:

◆ Nearly 60 million Americans have some form of heart or blood vessel disease.

◆ Cardiovascular disease accounted for about 41 percent of all deaths in 1997, the most recent year for which data are available.

◆ Cardiovascular disease kills more than half a million women each year—more than the next 14 causes of death combined.

◆ Among non-Hispanic blacks, 41 percent of men and 40 percent of women have some form of cardiovascular disease.

◆ Cardiovascular disease is the leading cause of death in African Americans, causing 37 percent of deaths among our population each year. Cancer comes in a close second, at 22 percent.

◆ Mortality rates for African American women are higher than any other racial or ethnic group for nearly every major cause of death including heart disease, lung cancer, breast cancer, and chronic obstructive pulmonary diseases.

◆ The rate of high blood pressure among blacks is among the highest in the world.

◆ 2.8 million African Americans have diabetes, and it is the fifth leading cause of death among all women and the sixth leading cause among all men.

◆ The prevalence of diabetes in African American women is approximately 85 percent higher than in Caucasian women.

◆ Black Americans are twice as likely to have diabetes as white Americans.

◆ Compared to whites, young African Americans have a two- to threefold greater risk of ischemic stroke, in which a blood vessel in the brain becomes blocked.

So watch your diet, folks!

Know Your Lean Mass

Before you can follow the upcoming dietary recommendations for your body type, you'll need to know how many pounds of lean mass you have (lean mass is your weight if you had no fat in your body at all). In order to figure out your lean mass, you'll need three things: a scale for determining your weight, a tape measure and a calculator. Once you've got these items, use the following guidelines:

Food Facts

As mentioned in Chapter 2, foods are composed of three basic elements: proteins, carbohydrates, and fats. Contrary to the teachings of today's trendy diets, you need *all* of these elements to maintain a fit, healthy body. Let me repeat: you need *all* these elements—protein, fat, and carbohydrates—to be healthy and look and feel great.

Let's take a brief look at each nutrient and the functions it performs in your body. Some of this might get slightly technical, but it's your body, so take responsibility. Read it, learn it, and then pass it on to your loved ones!

Protein. Protein is broken down by the body into amino acids, the "building blocks of muscle," which work to repair and rebuild muscle tissue, grow hair and nails, create enzymes and hormones, and maintain the health of your internal organs and blood. If you don't eat enough protein, you're going to be short on amino acids, and you're going to have a really hard time recovering from your workouts and building that calorie-burning muscle tissue.

But not all proteins are created equal, and high-fat options such as pork and ground beef are poor choices if you're looking to lose weight. Tuna, flank steak, skinless chicken breasts, egg whites, and lean turkey products are smarter options, as they're lower in fat and cholesterol and will work for you rather than against you. Vegetarian protein sources such as beans, nuts, tofu, and other soy products are okay, but often contain high amounts of fat and carbohydrates. So be careful when choosing these items for your meals. Read the labels when shopping! And check out the list of healthy protein sources below.

Fat. This element has gotten a bum rap for years, and people mistakenly think they should eliminate fat from their diets to lose weight. True, many people consume too much fat, leading to weight gain and obesity. But while most of us

FOR MEN

Before you use the formula, two measurements are required:
1. Body weight
2. Waist (measured at the belly button)

The equation:
1. (Body weight X 1.082) + 94.42 = Result 1
2. Result 1 – (waist girth X 4.15) = lean body mass

Example:
A professional male bodybuilder weighs 190 and has a 30¹/2-inch waist. Step 1: (190 X 1.082) + 94.42 = 300.
Step 2: 300 – (30.5 X 4.15) = 173.425 lbs

FOR WOMEN

Before you use the formula, five measurements are required:
1. Body weight
2. Wrist circumference (measured at the widest point)
3. Waist circumference (measured at the belly button)
4. Hip circumference (measured at the widest point)
5. Forearm circumference (measured at the widest point)

The equation:
1. Body weight X .0732 = Result 1
2. Result 1 + 8.987 = Result 2
3. Wrist ÷ 3.14 = Result 3
4. Waist X 0.157 = Result 4
5. Hip X 0.249 = Result 5
6. Forearm X 0.434 = Result 6
7. Result 2 + Result 3 = Result 7
8. Result 7 – Result 4 = Result 8
9. Result 8 – Result 5 = Result 9
10. Result 6 + Result 9 = lean body mass

Example:
A woman who weighs 125 pounds, and has a wrist measurement of 6.0, a waist measurement of 24 inches, a hip measurement of 38 inches, and a forearm measurement of 9.5 inches would calculate her body fat percentage in the following manner:
Step 1: 125 X 0.732 = 91.5
Step 2: 91.5 + 8.987 = 100.487
Step 3: 6 ÷ 3.14 = 1.91
Step 4: 24 X 0.157 = 3.768
Step 5: 38 X 0.249 = 4.123
Step 6: 9.5 X 0.434 = 4.123
Step 7: 100.487 + 1.91 = 102.397
Step 8: 102.397 – 3.768 = 98.629
Step 9: 98.629 – 9.462 = 89.167
Step 10: 4.123 + 89.167 = 93.29 lbs

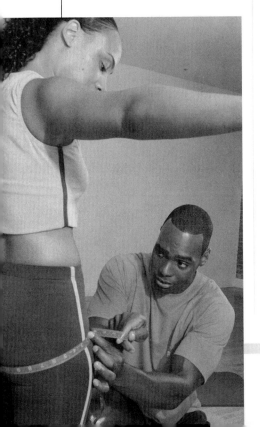

FOOD	SERVING SIZE	PROTEIN [GRAMS PER SERVING]
Very Lean Protein Sources		
Turkey or chicken breast, skinless	4 slices	20
Fish fillet (flounder, sole, scrod, cod, etc.)	1 fillet	41
Canned tuna in water	1 can	42
Shellfish (clams, lobster, scallop, shrimp)	1 cup	30
Cottage cheese, nonfat or low-fat	1 cup	28
Egg whites	2 large	7
Egg substitute	3 ounces	11
Beans, cooked (black, kidney, lentils, etc.)	1 cup	14
Lean Protein Sources		
Chicken, dark meat (skinless)	1/2 chicken	37
Turkey, dark meat (skinless)	1 cup	40
Salmon, swordfish, herring	1/2 fillet	32
Lean beef (flank steak, tenderloin, etc.)	3 ounces	24
Veal, roast or lean chop	3 ounces	23
Lamb, roast or lean chop	3 ounces	23
Pork, tenderloin or fresh ham	3 ounces	23
Low-fat luncheon meats	2 ounces	14
4.5% cottage cheese	1 cup	26
Sardines	1 can	22

need to cut back a lot on our fat intake, eliminating it completely is a mistake. Dietary fat is broken down by the body into fatty acids, which carry fat-soluble vitamins, create sex hormones, and contribute to the health of skin, eyes, nails, and hair.

There are two kinds of dietary fat: saturated and unsaturated. Saturated fat works negatively in your body, elevating cholesterol, clogging arteries and contributing to heart disease and obesity. These fats are found in palm oils, fatty

Dispelling the Myths

Myth 1: When you work out, fat turns into muscle.
Muscle and fat are two completely different substances, and one cannot create or be changed into the other. True, the body burns fat if you have a greater amount of lean mass and work out often, but it is never "changed into" muscle, although it might seem that way visually as you become leaner. The only way to get rid of body fat is through consistent exercise and a healthful, clean diet regimen.

Myth 2: If you eat fat, you will get fat.
This is both true and false. Eating an excess of any nutrient, including fat, can contribute to weight gain. But dietary fat is not the same as body fat, and although it might seem like that candy bar goes straight to your hips an hour after you eat it, things just don't work that way.

Myth 3: If your scale weight is high, you are fat.
The scale is a highly inaccurate measure of your fitness level, as it only measures how hard the earth is pulling you toward its center. As you begin to train with weights, your scale weight may initially go up, as muscle tissue (lean body mass) weighs about 75 percent more than fat. Even though you're increasing your body *weight,* you're likely lowering your body *fat* and are really getting smaller! So throw out that scale and go by how you look and how your clothes are fitting instead. If a particular pair of pants was tight when you began your program, and two weeks later the waistband feels loose, you're headed in the right direction.

Myth 4: The best way to lose weight is to skip meals.
Initially, you'll probably lose a few pounds if you stop eating or cut back your food intake drastically, but after a few days, your body gets wise to your plan and will go into "survival mode," storing anything and everything you put into your mouth as body fat. The best way to lose body fat is by following the diet outlined in this chapter and pairing it with a consistent exercise program.

Myth 5: People on carb-free diets lose 10 pounds of fat in one week!
People who cut their carbs do lose 10 pounds in their first week of dieting, but most of it is water. Your cells hold water inside of them to help metabolize carbohydrates, and when you eliminate carbs from your diet, your cells release this water, and you literally piss away 10 pounds. The only way to burn body fat is the slow, diligent, and safe way we've outlined here for you. Be in it for the long haul. Set yourself up to win.

meats, butter, margarine, and cheese—the bad stuff that tastes good. Unsaturated fat, on the other hand, can actually help lower cholesterol and is found in olive oil, nuts, even peanut butter—the good stuff that tastes good. All fats are a great source of energy, and a little bit can go a long way in terms of curbing hunger and alleviating sugar cravings.

Carbohydrates. These are probably the most misunderstood of all the nutrients, due in great part to the latest diets, like Atkins, that advocate low- or no-carb eating plans. But you absolutely need carbohydrates in order to perform your best, both physically and mentally, throughout the day. The type of carbs you eat, and when you eat them, has a lot to do with getting that hip-hop hard body.

When ingested, carbohydrates are broken down into simple sugars, or glucose, and are either used by the body right then and there for energy or stored in the muscles and the liver as glycogen. When your body runs out of ready glucose and glycogen, it begins to use protein from your muscles to fuel its daily functions. To avoid this catabolic state and keep from eating your muscles for breakfast, you need to have a steady intake of carbohydrates in your diet. There is a saying: "Fat burns in the flame of carbohydrates." This means that when you have enough carbs in your system, your body will use fat for fueling daily functions and activities instead of muscle tissue.

That being said, however, the carb choices you make are very important when trying to lose weight and get lean. To understand the kinds of carbs available, when to eat them and why, you have to understand the glycemic index. Now stay with me, because this can get technical, but it's essential to understand in order to further your weight-loss goals and get that sculpted shape.

The Glycemic Response and the Glycemic Index

Glycemic response is a technical term used to describe the measure of a particular food's ability to elevate blood sugar. Doctors have used it for years to help control blood-sugar levels in diabetic patients. When you eat a carbohydrate, your pancreas releases a hormone called insulin, which works to store nutrients to be used later for energy. But this hormone is a double-edged sword for people trying to lose weight. On the one hand, insulin is anabolic, meaning it

The Glycemic Index

HIGH GLYCEMIC FOODS	MODERATELY GLYCEMIC FOODS	LOW GLYCEMIC FOODS
Baked potato 85	Orange juice 57	Apple 36
Corn flakes 84	White rice 56	Pear 36
Cheerios 74	Popcorn 55	Skim milk 32
Graham crackers 74	Corn 55	Green beans 30
Honey 73	Brown rice 55	Lentils 29
Watermelon 72	Sweet potato 54	Kidney beans 27
White bread/bagel 70	Banana 50	Grapefruit 25
Raisins 65	Orange 43	Barley 25
Table sugar 64	Apple juice 41	

helps build and maintain lean muscle mass by driving protein substrates into your cells. On the other hand, it helps the body store excess calories as body fat—bad news if you're trying to lose weight. So how do you keep your body from storing fat and encourage it to make muscle? Follow the glycemic index for your carb choices. Don't worry, there's one in this chapter—I told you I got you!

The glycemic index rates foods according to their glycemic response. Foods with a high score are quickly broken down into glucose, elevating blood sugar immediately. (Remember: The higher your blood sugar, the higher your level of secreted insulin and the greater the potential for the ingested nutrients to be stored as body fat!) These high-glycemic, or "simple," carbs are usually processed food products that contain little fiber and often have added sugar, such as pasta, white breads, candy bars, and cereals.

Conversely, carbohydrates with a lesser number on the glycemic index, take longer to digest, elevate blood sugar to a lesser degree, and keep insulin production to a minimum. These "complex" carbohydrates are usually unprocessed whole foods with lots of fiber such as brown rice, fibrous vegetables, and sweet potatoes.

Choosing your carbohydrates wisely throughout the day will make a huge difference in both your energy level and your results. Low and moderately glycemic carbohydrates are best eaten early in the day and before exercise, since they provide sustained energy and help maintain stable blood-sugar levels. Higher glycemic carbs are great to consume immediately after exercise because they enter the bloodstream quickly and are readily available to fuel exercising muscles and repair them after the workout.

Feeding Frenzy

Now it's time to put this info to use and put together your diet. Remember, this "diet" is not a fad or a passing trend where you drink only grapefruit juice for the rest of your life. It's a lifestyle choice—a choice to be healthy and happy on the inside and out. A choice you'll make with every meal, every day, to maintain your lean, healthy hard body. Nutrition isn't rocket science. It's just a matter of being methodical and determined to make consciously healthful food choices that will benefit your body and mind each and every day.

Get hard-core with your nutrition and you'll have abs like LL's in no time! Memorize these tips and then start your campaign for a new you.

1. Captain's Log: Entries Made About Project Hip-Hop Hard Body. The first step is to identify what you're eating *right now*. While this might sound obvious, my clients are always shocked to learn what they actually eat on any given day. To help identify and clarify your eating habits, take two weeks and log everything—*everything*—that passes through your lips, from a sip of soda to a slice of pie to a Hershey's Kiss. You'll be surprised at how many additional calories you take in without realizing it. Also write down how you feel, what you did, and what happened to you on any given day. This will help you identify good and bad eating trends, as well as any emotional eating habits you might have and what triggers them. Continue using this journal in the coming weeks as you change your diet, habits, and body. It's great to be able to look back and see just how far you've come!

2. Cut the Crap. Eliminate any and all junk food from your diet. This includes any fast foods, processed lunch meats, chips, alcoholic beverages, sugared sodas, and all kinds of candy. You'll find that this one simple change will

Ch-Eating Out

Eating out can turn into a dietary nightmare
if you're not careful. Many supposedly "healthy" dishes in restaurants are exactly the opposite, containing hidden fat, sodium, and calories in sauces, dressings, or the preparation process. Ask for your dishes to be served dry, grilled, or broiled instead of sautéed, breaded, braised, or fried. Always ask for the sauce or salad dressing on the side so you control your fat intake instead of the chef. Replace heavy starch items such as mashed potatoes with grilled or steamed vegetables or a light salad.

Also, beware of overblown restaurant portions. Most restaurants consider a "single" serving to be a vat of pasta or a gallon of soup. Here's a great trick: up front, ask for a to-go box, and immediately put half your food into it and close the lid. Out of sight, out of mind, right? You'll be less tempted to eat it if it's not on your plate, and you have a tasty meal to look forward to later! Show some self-control. Eat to live, don't live to eat.

make a drastic difference in your energy, and you'll feel lighter, less bloated, and less moody.

3. Feed Frequently. Next, your goal is to lose weight by eating more. This may sound backward, but eating smaller meals more frequently throughout the day will keep your blood sugar stable and your stomach full, dispelling the urge to binge on junk food and preventing your body from becoming catabolic. It will also increase your metabolic rate, as your body is continually working to process nutrients, expel wastes, and build muscle. So if you usually eat three times a day, cut each meal in half and have six smaller meals and snacks instead. You'll still be having the same number of calories, but you'll be spreading them across the day. Your body is better able to deal immediately with smaller amounts of food, and will be less likely to store 300 to 400 calories of fat as it would be if you ate 1,000 calories all at once.

4. Slow and Steady. It might take some time to get used to eating six meals a day, so start slowly. First, learn to eat breakfast. Your body has been fasting for 8 to 10 hours while you were sleeping and needs some fuel to run right off the bat. Next, add a snack or small meal into your usual three-squares-daily in the midafternoon hours when people usually "crash." After a few weeks, add in another meal between breakfast and lunch, and finally a sixth one right after your workout. Eventually, your body will get used to having continual nourishment and you'll actually *want* to eat every 2 to 3 hours, but don't be afraid of this—this is good! It means your metabolism is speeding up and you're in need of more nutrients to maintain the lean, fat-burning machine that your body has become.

5. Trim the Fat. In order to lose body fat successfully, you must take in fewer calories than you expend. While this sounds simple in theory, it can be more difficult in practice, as 1 pound of fat is equal to 3,500 calories. Here's a good time to go back to your journal. Take a look at your eating habits and see where you can cut a few hundred calories here and there. If you can shave off a mere 350 calories per day, you'll lose a pound of fat in just 10 days! Add to that a regular exercise routine, and the pounds will melt away.

6. Manipulation and Regulation. As you become more adept at formulating your meals and better at gauging your energy levels, try experimenting with your carbs. Try eating higher glycemic items after your workout to encourage muscle repair and rebuilding. Eat starchy carbs (potatoes, rice, oatmeal) in your earlier meals, and have vegetables (broccoli, asparagus, spinach) later in the day to encourage fat burning instead of fat storage while you sleep. This will accelerate your body-fat loss over the long term so you can keep that hard body.

7. Water Your Waistline. Water aids in digestion, carries away the waste products of cells, and hastens recovery from workouts. Shoot for 8 to 10 glasses to begin with, increasing it to 1 liter, then 2 to 3 liters daily as your body cleans out and shapes up. Buy a water bottle and sip on it frequently at work, in the car, and during your workouts. After a few weeks, you'll never believe you survived without it! You can really feel the difference. Remember you have 60 days to do the job!

The Guidelines

Having read Chapter 2, you should know whether you're an ectomorph, a mesomorph, or an endomorph. Now that you know your lean mass as well, follow the specific recommendations below for your body type to determine the amounts of protein and carbohydrate food you should consume each day.

ENDOMORPH	ECTOMORPH	MESOMORPH
Protein: 1 gram of protein (lean) per 1 pound of lean body mass	*Protein:* 2 grams of protein (lean) per 1 pound of lean body mass	*Protein:* 2 grams of protein (lean) per 1 pound of lean body mass
Carbohydrate: 0.45 gram of carbohydrate (low-glycemic) per 1 pound of lean body mass	*Carbohydrate:* 3 grams of carbohydrate per 1 pound of lean body mass	*Carbohydrate:* 1.5 grams of carbohydrate per 1 pound of lean body mass
Example: An endomorph man with a lean body mass of 166 pounds should eat 166 grams of protein (1 gram x 166) and 75 grams of carbohydrate (0.45 x 166) daily.		

Let Them Eat Cake!

Of course, people gotta live, and I don't expect you to be a complete saint! As I mentioned in Chapter 2, I'm a huge advocate of "cheating": having one meal a week where you eat something you've been craving or dreaming about that's not in your diet plan. Allowing yourself a desired food item can help alleviate the need and craving for it, and it will help you stick to your diet during the next week. But once you've gotten it out of your system, go right back to eating the righteous way.

I do not advocate, however, rewarding yourself with food for reaching certain goals. This creates a negative relationship with food and can become detrimental to you mentally and physically in the long run. So instead of bingeing on cheesecake when you make partner in your law firm or break 135 on the scale, treat yourself to something other than food.

DAILY MENU PLAN

Using the preceding example of the endomorphic man with a lean body mass of 166 pounds, the following is a sample menu plan for one day that would meet his requirements. *This is only a sample.* Use your own imagination and personal preferences in planning your own meals or in choosing appropriate meals in a restaurant:

FOOD	SERVING SIZE (GRAMS/SERVING)	CARBS (GRAMS/ SERVING)	PROTEIN (GRAMS/ SERVING)
Breakfast			
Grapefruit	1/2 fruit (120 g)	11	3
Cottage cheese (nonfat)	1 cup (226 g)	6	28
Turkey bacon	3 servings (42 g)	0	6
Coffee	1 cup	0	0
Subtotal		**17**	**37**
Mid morning snack			
Pear	1 small (120 g)	1	0
Protein shake	2 scoops powder	2	17
Subtotal		**13**	**17**
Lunch			
Canned tuna in water	1 can (165 g)	0	42
Tossed green salad	1 1/2 cup (207 g)	6	2
Light mayonnaise	1 tbsp (15 g)	1	0
Subtotal		**7**	**44**

FOOD	SERVING SIZE (GRAMS/SERVING)	CARBS (GRAMS/ SERVING)	PROTEIN (GRAMS/ SERVING)
Mid afternoon snack			
Almonds, dry roasted	20 kernels	5	6
Subtotal		**5**	**6**
Dinner			
Fish fillet	1 fillet (180 g)	0	41
Sweet potato	1/2 medium (75 g)	14	1
Asparagus	8 spears (120 g)	5	3
Soy sauce	1 tsp	0	0
Subtotal		**19**	**45**
Bedtime snack			
Popcorn	1 cup	8	0
Beef jerky	2 pieces (40 g)	4	13
Subtotal		**12**	**13**
Total		**73**	**162**

Fitting It All In

I'm sure this sounds a bit overwhelming, and it will take a little getting used to. But believe me, you'll soon become an expert at planning your meals and regulating your nutritional needs. As your body becomes healthier and toxin-free, you'll feel lighter, freer, and inspired to continue and move forward.

Make this clean, healthful eating plan your *new* soul food. This is a lifetime commitment; an investment in your body, mind, and spirit; an insurance policy better than any you can buy. Eat well, live well, and be a participant in life.

How to Get Abs Like D'Angelo

When D'Angelo filmed the video for his 2000 hit Untitled (How Does It Feel), he bared a lot more than his soul on camera. Had the director panned another inch or two below D's ripped midsection, fans would have been measuring him against porn stars, not pro athletes.

Believe it or not, four months before that shoot, D was so badly out of shape and so uncomfortable that at first he wouldn't even take off his shirt with me. I said, "Dude, I need to see what your body looks like." I didn't actually get a look until 30 days into our sessions, and only after D started getting results. We must have done okay, because now half the women in the audience throw their panties at him when he walks on stage.

The trick was stripping away the layers of fat that had buried his ab muscles. You can train your abs all day long, but if you don't follow a sensible diet and perform regular aerobic exercise, you're not going to see them. I've seen lots of fat people with hard stomachs. So I dieted him down to lean him out. I had him eat three food meals a day along with drinking three protein shakes, and we timed them so that he was constantly tapping into his fat stores.

As for ab training, I had him do a lot of weighted stuff to carve him out a deep six-pack. We didn't try to make his stomach flat. We tried to build his abs up so they would protrude more—bodybuilder abs, as opposed to fitness-model abs. If you want to achieve the same look, add an extra session or two of core training to your regimen each week. (Together, your abs and lower back are referred to as your *core*.)

Here's how you can get the same look: Take five or six ab exercises—feel free to use the ones in Chapters 2 and 4—and arrange them as a circuit. That means you do maybe 30 reps of the first exercise, rest only long enough to gulp some water, and continue that way until you've completed all the exercises. At that pace, it shouldn't take more than 8 to 10 minutes to go the whole nine. If you have enough stamina to repeat the circuit, go for it. If you can't, make that your goal. Better yet, add some resistance to your ab exercises. Weighted leg raises, weighted crunches on an exercise ball, medicine tosses on the ball—stuff like that will really make your abs pop.

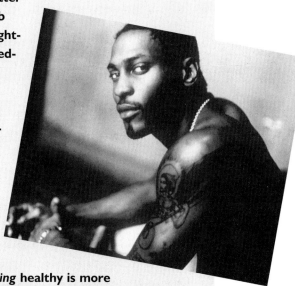

One other secret to D's amazing success was that we didn't neglect his lower back. In fact, if I had to work one or the other, I would choose the lower back, using deadlifts and reverse hyperextensions. In most people, the lower back isn't as strong as the abs, and if that imbalance persists, an injury will follow. Remember, *being* healthy is more important than *looking* healthy. Work your abs and lower back.

Was the effort D put in worth it? I would argue that it was the best career move he's ever made. Musicians need diesel bodies for more than just looking good. When it comes time to go on tour, the better shape they're in, the longer they can go, and the better their performances will be—all of which can translate into some major bank!

D is one of my favorite clients because he pushes hard. The proof is in the ripped-abs trend you see all over the place. Who do you think started it?

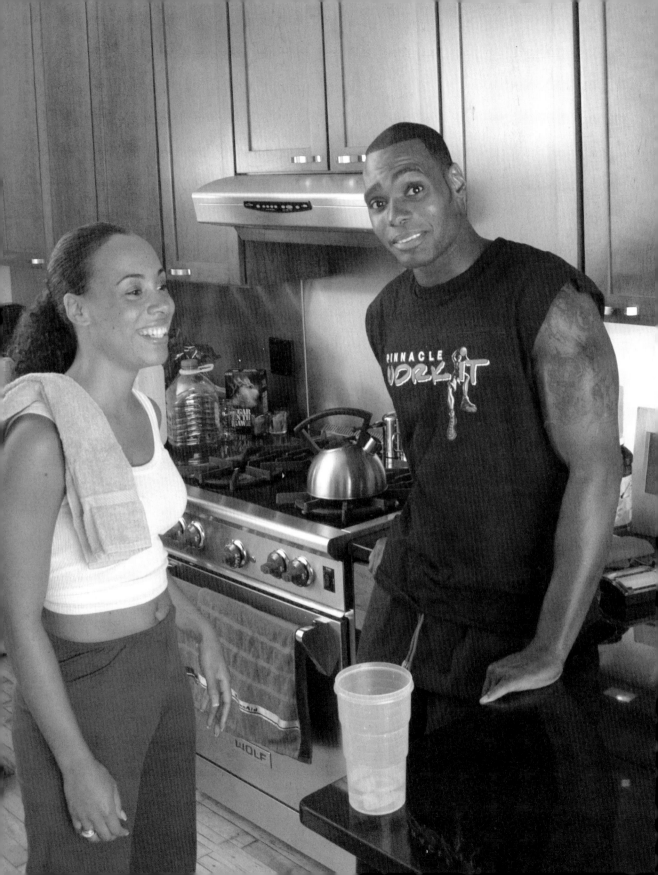

The 411 on Fitness FAQs

Fat Loss and Breast Size

Q: I've been losing weight for the past year, which is great, but my breasts have gotten smaller, too, which isn't so great. Short of getting implants, is there anything I can do?

A: Not knowing more in the way of specifics about your body-fat levels, that's a hard question for me to answer. But if you chronically undereat for your body size and activity level, that could affect your breast size. Women in particular have been so conditioned by chronic dieting that they think 1,200 calories a day is sufficient, no matter how many calories they burn. In reality, even 1,500 calories could be insufficient if you're training hard and working around the clock.

Eat according to your activity level—you might need more food to fill out. Regarding training, you can also accentuate your upper pec muscles with exercises like incline bench presses. Building the muscle underneath will give you fuller-looking breasts.

Also, some of my female clients have told me that breast fullness improves when they supplement with essential fatty acids. More on those in the nutrition chapter.

To Eat or Not to Eat

Q: If I do my cardio in the morning, is it better to eat or not eat before doing so, assuming burning fat is my goal?

A: You hear a ton of opinions on this one, both pro and con, but it makes little difference at day's end. Meal timing has some small effects on how the body uses its energy stores, but the big-picture items, like your overall diet and exercise consistency, really make the difference.

The big controversy here is that although you might tap into your fat stores more by doing cardio on an empty stomach, you might not have enough energy to have a good workout. It's highly individualized. Some people can do it and have a great workout and push through it, but other people get so depleted that it's not worth it.

This is one of those questions that an expert can't answer hard-and-fast for you. You have to experiment. It's really a matter of knowing your own body, and that's going to take time.

Picture This

Q: I've thought about getting a tattoo and navel piercing, and if I proceed, I want to make sure I do it in a way that eliminates the risk of contracting hepatitis—or anything else, for that matter. Any suggestions?

A: Okay, I see that you noticed that I have a tattoo and a nipple ring—which I got on a dare from my wife!

Even if all your friends get a tattoo, don't do it impulsively or without forethought. First, talk to those friends who've gotten one, and ask them if they would do it again, and how they would have done it differently.

If you decide to take the plunge, look for an artist whose work you like, and then check out his or her studio. Tattoos and piercings produce small amounts of bleeding, which puts you at risk of contracting hepatitis B and C. The studio should be clean and hygienic. Look for needle sterilizers and other sanitary equipment. Many states have health regulations for body art, so if the shop, artist, or both are licensed, look for the posting and date of the permit or permits.

Think long and hard, too, about where the image is going to reside on your body. You may think having Prince's symbol stamped on both wrists looks amazing, but your employer may be far less enamored of it, consigning you to a business wardrobe of long-sleeve shirts exclusively. A better location might be one more easily obscured by clothing.

Finally, be prepared for the aftercare that tattoos and piercings require. You need to care for these wounds as long as they remain open, particularly in areas vulnerable to infection, like the navel and the rim of the ear.

By the way, I got my stuff done at Tattoo Mania on the Sunset Strip in Cali.

Start Fast

Q: I'm trying to get my diet squared away, and I plan to start with break-fast. Because I don't have time to prepare, say, egg whites or protein pancakes at home, I've decided to eat a bowl of cereal each morning before leaving for work. With so many kinds to choose from, though, what should I be looking for?

A: Choose whole-grain cereals, which are loaded with vitamins and minerals, rather than Sugar Smacks, Count Chocula, and other cereals that are sweetened with processed sugar, much like candy. To avoid that, make sure sugar isn't among the first three ingredients listed on the package. Also, look for a cereal that contains 4 to 5 grams of fiber per serving.

One hundred percent bran is a good choice, also oatmeal, and hot cereals, which contain really good grains. There are also flax seed cereals, which are incredible. These are a great way to start your day because they're an extremely good source of energy from carbohydrate. There are even some studies suggesting that people who eat oatmeal have a lower risk of heart disease than those who don't. Pour low-fat or skim milk onto any of these cereals and add a good source of protein and calcium to the mix. Or throw a scoop of whey protein on there for a complete meal.

Tale of the Tape

Q: I'm about to start the Jump Off. So I'm hyped up about embarking on a new exercise routine and diet that will help me shed the extra weight I've accumulated over the past five years of relative inactivity. However, I'm not sure how I should measure my progress. Should I just weigh myself every day?

A: No! Do not put that kind of pressure on yourself. Use the mirror and be consistent. You should weigh yourself once every two weeks. And you shouldn't be alarmed if you're not losing weight, as long as you see changes visually. You're probably replacing fat with muscle in that case. As long as you're losing inches, don't sweat it.

Head Game

Q: I try sticking with my training, but I throw in the towel as soon as I miss one or two workouts, in part because I'm a perfectionist with an all-or-nothing approach to most activities. Is there anything I can do to overcome this chronic tendency?

A: The best thing you can do is to keep going to the gym. There's no way to get around it. You have to understand that the commitment is long-term. You're going to make mistakes, and if you fall off the wagon, get right back on. The most successful people fail a lot, but they just get back up and try again. Don't quit completely because you stumble. Get back on it.

Glute Salute

Q: I've heard that doing plié squats are great for firming up my glutes, but I have trouble keeping my back straight with my feet in that position. Help!

A: Try performing them using a Smith machine or with a stability ball against a wall. The Smith in particular allows you to keep your feet in a wide, turned-out stance in front of your body, and it allows you to keep your back straight as you descend. It's a short range of motion, but if you keep your glutes contracted throughout, you'll see major results. Pulse up and down slowly. Do sets of 30 or 40. You tough guys can even hold dumbbells.

Hip-Hop Stink-Body

Q: When I do any sort of cardio or aerobics class, I sweat really badly. Toweling myself off interrupts my workouts, and sometimes I even slip on the dripping sweat. My mom says that when you sweat it means you're healthy; I wonder if it means I'm out of shape, or if it might even be indicative of an underlying medical problem. What do you think?

A: It doesn't sound like a medical problem. Heavy sweating usually means your body is efficient at cooling itself, which is a good thing. Headbands and wristbands can help absorb some of the moisture. I'm a heavy sweater as well, so I wear one shirt and bring another to change into halfway through. Heavy-duty deodorant is also a good idea—the other gym patrons will thank you. If you really think you're problem is more serious, though, definitely consult a doctor.

Ten the Easy Way

Q: I never used to have a weight problem, but now, at 29, I find myself with 10 extra pounds that I just can't seem to shake. What's the first thing I should do to correct this problem?

A: This happens to everyone. Your metabolism is slowing down at the same time that your activity level is slowing down. Work has probably become very important, and your forms of entertainment have probably become seated ones: restaurants, business dinners, lunches—shopping at the mall instead of playing football like in the good old days of your youth. You just can't eat the same as you did back when you were superactive. However, high-intensity exercises can offset that and burn a lot of those calories that would otherwise be stored as body fat. Ten pounds is not that far off. Train and eat right. No more coasting!

Know Thine Enemy

Q: I've managed to adhere to my diet for three months, and even when I go out to eat, I'm able to stick with the program, more or less. "Less" concerns the buffet line, where I tend to overeat still. I really don't know what I should be putting on my plate and what I should be avoiding. Help!

A: As a general principle, try to eat a handful of each serving. But this is another one of those individualized questions that falls in the realm of: Be true to and honest with yourself. For example, has your day's energy expenditure justified going back for seconds?

Buffet lines don't have to be a nutritional disaster area. In fact, because they offer so much variety, buffets can be great for fit, health-conscious people if they know what they're doing. Get a salad, and then put egg whites and turkey on it, and maybe some fish, and suddenly you've got a nice combination of lean protein and carbs. The key is educating yourself about the caloric content and nutritional value of foods—and that's something you should be doing anyway!

The See-Food Diet?

Q: I read in some diet book that when I crave something, my brain is actually telling my body what it needs. Does this mean I can eat whatever I want whenever I want without compromising my health and fitness?

A: In a word, no. If that were true, people would be craving milk, because they probably need more calcium; or spinach, because they probably need more folic acid; or whole grains, instead of doughnuts, cake, and soda. Cravings tend to be more situational and emotional. In the midst of our hectic lives, we lose touch with what true hunger is. Instead, we rely on external cues, like walking past a fast-food restaurant at noon thinking, That's what I need for lunch—when in fact you don't. Or thinking, Having that hot chocolate will make me feel better. Think about it. Don't be an emotional eater.

The Skinny on Aerobics and Fat Burning

Q: Do lower-intensity activities such as walking or low-impact aerobics really burn more fat than higher-intensity activities?

A: Good question. It's true that a higher percentage of calories used for energy during low-intensity exercise come from fat, but in absolute terms, you'll burn more fat calories, as well as more of all the other kinds of calories, with a high-intensity workout. One person may work out for an hour on a treadmill at low intensity and burn a hypothetical 300 calories total; about 200 of those come from fat. Another person training as hard as she can might burn 600 calories, with 250 coming from fat. Since losing a pound of fat requires a total deficit of 3,500 calories, you'll get there faster with higher-intensity workouts. These workouts will also keep your heart rate elevated beyond the scope of the session, which means more fat burning for you.

The Long Haul

Q: Everything in *The Jump Off* sounds nice and skippy, and I don't mean to be a hater, but how can I stay with this long-term?

A: As a motivational coach and personal trainer, I try to do my best to keep my clients motivated. Sometimes I win, sometimes I lose, but even if I win 95 percent of the time, there's always that 5 percent that I just can't turn around. I try my best to explain the benefits, I try my best to make it fun for them, and I try to make it innovative, but it doesn't always work.

The best way to stay focused is to make sure you get results from your training. Therefore, your training has to be as efficient as possible for you to get those results. It has to be worthwhile for you to do. Once you get in shape and you reach a goal, then you're no longer training to get results. That's the most difficult time to stay in shape, because the changes are less obvious. You're not getting that same excitement out of it.

Once you reach that level, the key is to change what your training goal is. Maybe it has to turn to more of a performance thing. For each person at each level of fitness, your motivation has to be different. For me personally, when I first started training and I was fat, I was so much more motivated going to the gym. Then it became my occupation, so I was doing it for more than just the love of getting my body in shape. I had to relearn to be enthusiastic about my own workouts. I learned how to run 20 miles at 230 pounds at a 7-minute-mile pace, and do 12 rounds with a heavy bag—athletic stuff. That and I got my wife into working out, which really helped, because it became an activity that we could enjoy together.

For this to work, you have to find the things that motivate you. Will yourself to succeed. This book is a spark—only you can turn it into a fire!

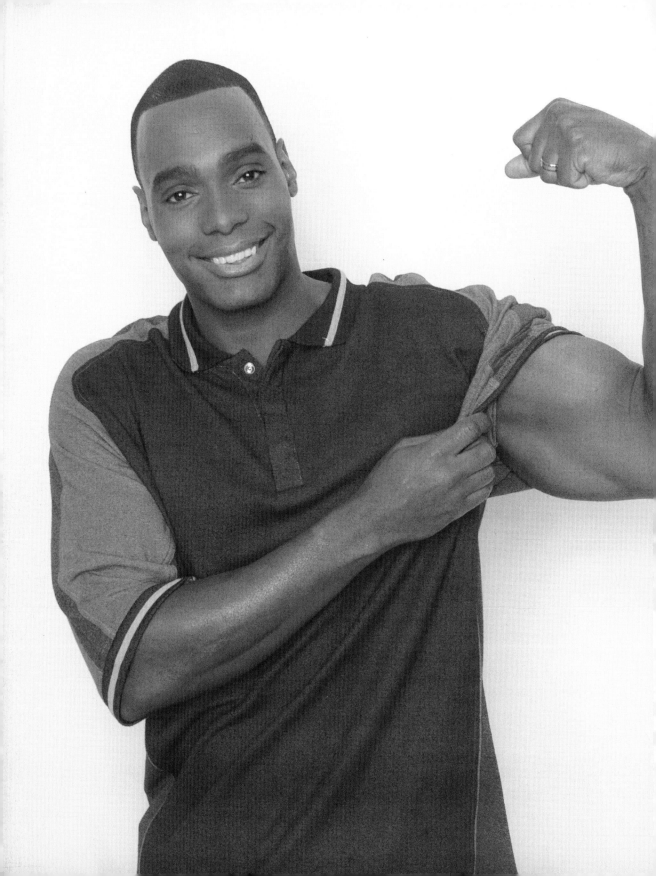

Aftermath

Now that you've read this book, I have one final jewel to drop on you: Success doesn't depend on reading this book. Seriously, I know that isn't what you expected to hear, but I want to separate myself from the rest of the fitness personalities out there by telling you the hard truth. This book does have fantastic workouts and a nutritional program based on university studies, but what does that mean if you're not motivated or inspired enough to push through the workouts and change your eating habits? As I said in the last chapter, what this book does provide is a spark. But you have to provide the fuel and fan the flames to fire yourself up enough to stay the course and change your life.

The book is a road map that can help you get to your destination, but you have to take that first step and make that leap of faith. And guess what? I believe you can do it.

Why? Because I'm just like you. I'm one of you. I'm a real person with real issues who took some steps to change my whole life. I'm not saying that your whole life will change instantly, but I have been in the training game for over 10 years, and I've seen it happen thousands of times. I've seen teenagers who smoke weed every day quit because they start to care about their bodies, I've trained teenage girls who will never have unprotected sex because they value their health now. I've seen overweight women get in shape and pass the FBI's boot camp because they believed in themselves. I saw P. Diddy run a marathon and Mary J. Blige change her life.

I've seen so many people change their story, and I know you can do it, too. Change your story and be like, *Damn, I can't eat this. I have to go to the gym today.* Get excited about taking steps toward self-improvement.

Stay in Control!

Unfortunately, while you try to lift yourself up, the player haters always try to break you down. Make no mistake: when people who once saw you in a certain light witness your transformation, inside and out, the player-hating will begin. A lot of people won't want you to get in shape because of their own agendas. Your boyfriend might *like* you feeling insecure about your body, because in that state he assumes you'll stay with him, no matter what he does or says. Your employer might *like* you being 50 pounds overweight, because if you lose that weight and your self-esteem rises, you just might demand that raise you know you deserve. Or you might go out and get a better job, one that better matches your true abilities.

Wouldn't it be nice to get some support once in a blue? But don't worry. These people have a preconceived idea of who you are and what your place should be, and it can intimidate them to see your story changing right in front of them. It makes them question themselves and where they will fit in your life. Your change forces them to look at themselves, and they may not be ready to do that. In turn, they may try to sabotage you, perhaps without even realizing what they're doing. So beware! Stay in control and don't buy into what they say, especially if they try to stick old labels on you. Remember, it's up you to define yourself, and part of that is not buying into how other people define you.

One way you can make sure to incorporate fitness into your lifestyle is by constantly reminding yourself of the payoff. Take control of your mind. If it's beginning to get difficult, tell yourself: *I am doing this to be a better me, to be around for my kids, for a better relationship with my mate, to have more energy and confidence, to improve my performance at work, and to be better, stronger, faster.* (I got that from the *Six-Million Dollar Man*.)

Another motivation can be to inspire others you care about to take their health seriously. You can't take care of others until you get yourself straight, which should motivate you to commit to improving yourself. Maybe it's your children, maybe it's your spouse, and maybe it's your belief in yourself. It's up to you to find the reasons closest to your heart that will keep you on the path and get you there as quickly as possible. Lead by example. Walk the walk.

Find the Excitement in Each Day

Once you've made this transformation, your whole approach to life will change. I can tell you from my personal experience that now, even though I set the alarm for six o'clock in the morning, I always get up at five. I'm just fired up about starting my day. (It's not like I hit the sack early, either. I'm often up training clients like Diddy, who's been known to work out at midnight or three in the morning.) My wife Natasha gets pissed because I wake up our daughter Skylar every time I get up, but I can't help it. I wish other people could find that excitement and joy in each day. Life is so great, but it's so short at the same time. Don't waste it.

Once you embrace the fitness lifestyle, you won't associate going to the gym with trudging off to work. You can force yourself to do that for a while, but it won't last for long. It has to be fun for you to be in it for the long term. Success comes when you can't wait to hit the weights. The same goes for dieting. Eventually you'll reach the point where you'll think the benefits you're getting from this are greater than the sacrifices you're making. That's the mind-set you need to make it work. In fact, at that point, you won't even be thinking about "diet" (which implies a temporary way of eating) as any different from your normal way of life.

Your decision making will change as well. You'll start saying, *Hey, let me buy this fitness magazine instead of buying that other thing that I really don't need*. Or instead of buying that 50-inch flat-screen TV, you'll cop the 40-inch instead, and use the leftover dough to pay for some private training sessions. The money is usually there; it's just a question of what you choose to spend it on. Most of us spend $100 on cable each month. It may seem like a necessity, but it's not. Your body, your health, and your life are the real necessities.

Another reason you won't view training and eating right as sacrifices is that you will have developed the wisdom to realize that the long-term cost of ignoring your body is huge. Heart disease, high blood pressure, diabetes, arthritis, back pain, bone deterioration, loss of income due to illness—all of these and more thrive in the absence of exercise and proper diet. And if the individual costs are alarming, the costs to society are mind-boggling. Our national health-care system is straining badly under the weight of this increased demand and shrinking resources, and the persistence of present trends could lead to its collapse. Worst of all, children, teens, and young adults are increasingly at risk. In a study published recently in the *Journal of the American Medical Association*, researchers from Stanford University found that many Mexican American and African American children, some as young as 9, are *already* developing risk factors for heart disease. I don't know about you, but I don't think a 9-year-old should be doomed to anything more unpleasant than homework—certainly not heart disease. It's a shame, because it's all preventable.

Life-threatening habits are forming at an alarming rate in other groups as well. For example, 16 percent of white teenage girls in the United States now smoke, and that's eight times higher than the rate for African American girls. The health crisis in the United States does not discriminate. We need to encourage youngsters to exercise more, eat junk food less, and quit smoking. Make sure you pass on to your children the gift of health and self-empowerment. For our children to realize their potential, they must keep their bodies as finely tuned as their minds. Of course, one feeds off the other: A good training regimen, followed consistently, builds mental stamina as effectively as it builds muscle, strength, and endurance. When this starts happening, society as a whole will benefit.

Fully appreciating each day is part of living in the moment, and that's another important aspect of making fitness a lifestyle. When you focus on the here and now, you make fewer mistakes. When you keep your eye on the ball, you don't drop it. Do the right thing now, and the future will take care of itself. Short-term focus produces achievable goals that lead to long-term success. Don't think, *Damn, I have to work out for the rest of my life!* Instead, try to take it one workout at a time. Don't think about dieting; think, *I'm just going to get this meal right at this time.* If you live in the moment, it's always easier.

Don't get me wrong. Long-term goals are incredibly important. These are the grand prizes that we're all after. But when you work backward from that goal of, say, losing 30 pounds, you realize that what you really need to focus on is taking care of tonight's workout and your next meal. In other words, instead of focusing on tighter glutes, focus on the small things you need to acquire them, like proper form when you squat and going hard on leg day.

Most people don't live in the moment. They live in the past or in the future. This is the mind-set I hate: *I have failed to get in shape in the past, so this time won't be any different.* Or, *I can't get in shape right now, but when I get some time (or money), then, world watch out!* They spend all their time dwelling on the failures of the past or daydreaming about the future instead of taking care of business in the present. But without hard work in the here and now, your history will repeat itself. So it is with all things. The way to achieve your goals is to step forward *in the moment.* If you want to change the way you look and live in the future, then the only way to do that is to get busy right now, in the present.

There are a couple of keys to this.

No matter how small the victory, celebrate it. Honor yourself for your accomplishment. You did an extra five minutes on the treadmill? Great. Think about how that takes you so much closer than five minutes to your goal. Imagine what you can do tomorrow. And the day after.

Build momentum. Get into a rhythm. Give yourself a pat on the back after every workout. I pat myself on the back even after a bad workout, because if you look at it philosophically, there's no such thing as a bad workout—at least you got the workout done. Maybe you didn't progress like you wanted to, but you didn't backslide, either. Think positive.

The same goes for nutrition. When you eat a healthy meal, think, *I did it!* With each victory you'll get closer to your ultimate goal. No matter how small the accomplishment, it's important to celebrate. Other people won't congratulate you, especially if health is a problem for them. Your girlfriend's not going to tell you you're getting into great shape when she's overweight. You have to do it for yourself. You deserve it! Help yourself and then help someone else. Pass it on!

The Path to Success

It's all about taking care of you so you can take better care of others. This means not getting overextended. There's a certain amount of selfishness you have to have, if only for self-preservation. That means not letting people take all your time so you can't even get in shape. You work hard, you train hard, and you need downtime for rest and relaxation. It's important for people to unwind. I push myself as hard as anyone you'll ever meet, but the reason I can do that is because I take care of my mind, my body, and my spirit. I take time out from the world to take care of myself.

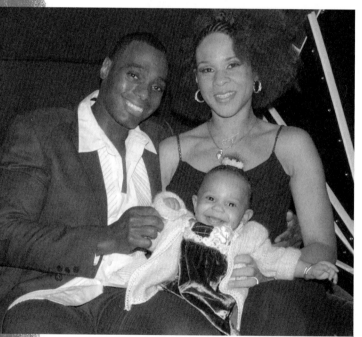

Out with the fam!

Something I've been doing religiously for years is taking a nap in the middle of the day. I shut it down for 45 minutes or an hour, regardless of where I am. If I'm driving in Manhattan, I just pull the car over someplace quiet, where's there's no traffic, and just shut it down. When my wife Natasha and I get up in the morning, the first thing we do is pray. It's all about staying grounded and finding that balance.

To enjoy the struggle, you need that downtime, so you can build yourself up with positive self-talk. That means you're rested and energized when it's time to attack. It's a rough world out there. You've got to psyche yourself up. Believe in what you're saying, or no one else will.

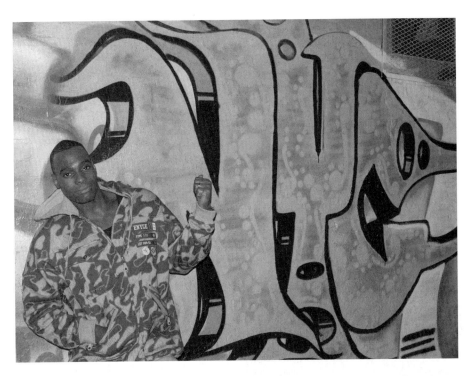

On the road to creating a better you, there are numerous exits and tempting detours, all designed to lead you astray from the path of self-improvement. There will be detours that offer instant gratification and pleasure, whether it's skipping that scheduled workout due to soreness or eating that slice of cheesecake, or a player-hating boyfriend or girlfriend taking you out for drinks when they knew you had to work out that night. But you must stay on the path to receive the ultimate rewards, a healthier you, and all the benefits that come with that. Remember, it's your body and it's your life—you can do it!

I hope I've been able to inspire you through these words, to take that first step and fight the good fight. I've certainly gained a lot of self-discovery by writing it, so I'd like to thank all of you for that. I tried to put all of my heart and soul into these words, to try and lead you to take action. I know you won't let me down. More importantly, I know you won't let yourself down. Train hard, live your life, and God bless. Peace one, baby.

—Mark Jenkins

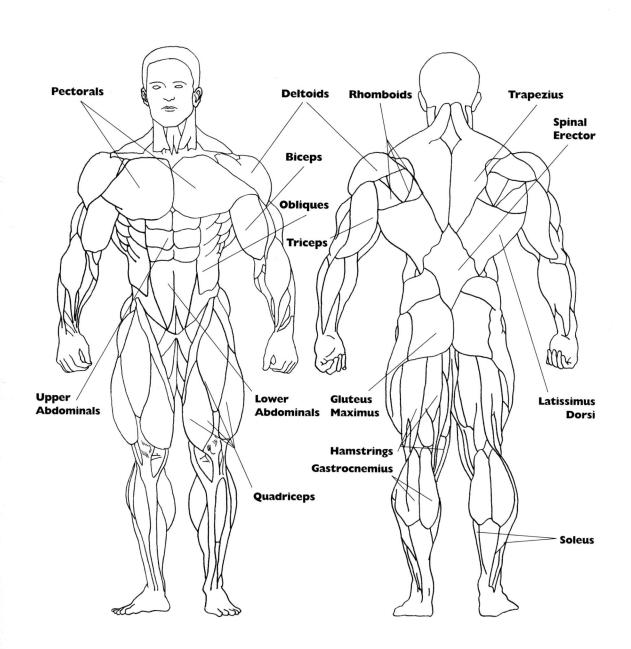

Pectorals

Deltoids   Rhomboids   Trapezius

Biceps   Spinal Erector

Obliques

Triceps

Upper Abdominals   Lower Abdominals   Gluteus Maximus   Latissimus Dorsi

Hamstrings

Gastrocnemius

Quadriceps   Soleus

Glossary

Adaptation: (also called "plateauing") when your body becomes used to an activity (cardiovascular or resistance) and stops making visible progress.

Aerobic Exercise: Means literally "with oxygen." Used to describe continual cardiovascular exercise in which oxygen is used to sustain the activity.

Amino Acids: The building blocks of protein. Utilized by the body to repair and rebuild muscle tissue.

Anabolic: A positive, internal physical state in which your body uses available nutrients to build and repair muscle tissues.

Anaerobic Exercise: Quick, intense bursts of energy in which oxygen in not utilized or needed. This occurs when sprinting, jumping, and other such intense, quick activities.

Ballistic Stretching: An unsafe, outdated flexibility technique in which the participant bounces explosively over an extended limb in order to force a muscle to elongate.

Bodyfat: (also called "adipose tissue") The stored calories held on your person in the form of fatty, subcutaneous tissue (read, saddlebags, spare tires, and love handles!)

Carbohydrates: The main dietary macronutrient that provides the body with energy when broken down into its smaller component, glucose.

Catabolic: A negative, internal physical state in which your body breaks down and utilizes muscle tissue (protein) for fuel in the absence of usable nutrients.

Cholesterol: An organic compound found in animal products, dairy products, and some oils that works negatively in the body to promote heart disease and obesity (when ingested in excessive amounts).

Complex Carbohydrates: Low glycemic foods that contain high amounts of fiber, such as oatmeal or brown rice, take a long time to break down and provide long-term, sustained energy for the body.

Concentric Phase: The part of an exercise repetition in which the muscle is contracting (shortening).

Core: The central part of your body that works to keep you upright, standing, and stable as well as allowing you to bend forward and back and side to side. Encompasses the abdominals, lower back, sides, and hip flexors.

Diabetes: A metabolic disease in which insulin production is inadequate for the regulation of normal blood glucose levels. Can be hereditary or dietary.

Dietary Fat: A high-energy macronutrient found in foods like nuts, meats, and oils that promote satiety, provide sustained energy, work to regulate hormones, transport fat-soluble vitamins, and maintain the health of skin, hair, and nails.

DOMS: Delayed Onset Muscle Soreness. The pain and stiffness you feel 24 to 48 hours after a workout. Caused by a buildup of lactic acid and other cellular wastes in the muscle tissues.

Eccentric Phase: The portion of an exercise repetition in which the muscle lengthens (elongates).

Ectomorph: A naturally thin person who has a delicate bone structure and lean musculature and a difficult time putting on weight.

Emotional Eating: A negative behavior in which food is used to ease an emotional pain such as anxiety, stress, or depression.

Empty Calories: A term used to describe foods that are nearly devoid of nutritional benefit, such as cola beverages or candy bars.

Endomorph: A large-boned, heavyset person who naturally tends to holds a lot of body fat and has an easy time gaining weight.

Endorphins: Natural feel-good substances produced by the brain during sustained exercise that promote feeling of well-being and happiness. It's nature's morphine!

Frequency: How often work is performed. Can mean the number of times you train in a week or the number of times you hit a particular body part per week.

Glucose: A simple sugar derived from the breakdown of carbohydrates that is used by the body and brain for energy.

Glycemic Index: A chart that rates foods according to their glycemic response. A high score indicates that a food is quickly broken down into glucose. A low score indicates a food is more slowly digested and assimilated.

Glycemic Response: The measure of a food's ability to elevate blood sugar.

Glycogen: Calories stored in the muscles and liver to be utilized for energy during aerobic activity.

Insulin: A hormone produced by the pancreas in response to carbohydrate intake. Works to metabolize carbs and fats by driving food substrates into cells either for use or for storage.

Intensity: The level of difficulty at which you perform an activity, whether it's cardio, strength training, or flexibility.

Interval Training: A mostly anaerobic cardiovascular training method in which periods of all-out, intensive exercise are interspersed with periods of less intense, working recovery.

Isometric Contraction: A muscle contraction in which the muscle contracts without changing its length and in which no joints move.

Lactic Acid: A byproduct of muscular activity, specifically the metabolism of carbs and glycogen in muscle cells, that causes soreness and stiffness (see DOMS).

Mesomorph: A midsized, medium-boned person who falls between an ectomorph and an endomorph, retaining a solid amount of muscle mass while remaining lean.

Metabolism: The chemical activity of a cell or tissue that transforms nutrients into energy.

Multijoint Exercise: An action involving movement around more than one joint or limb, such as a squat, a pull-up, or a push-up.

Overtraining: An exercise overdose that causes a breakdown in the recovery system of the body, usually resulting from excessive exercise, improper training, insufficient recovery, and poor nutrition.

Peak Contraction: The point during a repetition at which the muscles are fully, eccentrically contracted.

Reps (or Repetitions): The number of times an exercise is repeated to complete one set. One rep involves moving a weight from the start position, through the movement itself, and back to the start through a muscle's full range of motion.

Saturated Fats: (also called trans fats) A kind of dietary fat found in butter, mayonnaise, fried foods, and most desserts worth a damn. It is known to contribute to obesity, diabetes, and heart disease when eaten in excess.

Set: The number of times you repeat a sequence of repetitions for a single exercise.

Simple Carbs: Processed or refined foods such as white bread, fruit juice, or cola drinks, which are easily broken down into glucose and are quickly assimilated by the body.

Single-Joint Exercise: An exercise involving motion around only one joint, such as a biceps curl or a calf raise.

Spot Reduction: The myth that you can specifically work one part of the body in order to "burn" the fat off that particular area.

Static Stretching: A flexibility technique in which the participant strikes a stretching pose and holds it for 10 to 60 seconds, allowing the muscle to relax and elongate without bouncing or yanking.

Steady State: An aerobic cardiovascular technique in which the participant maintains a certain level of intensity for the duration of the workout.

Unsaturated Fat: A dietary fat found in foods like avocados, nuts, and olive oil that works positively in the body to promote good heart health, lower cholesterol and provide energy.

Visualization: A mental training technique in which a positive outcome is envisioned as the work is performed. For example, imagining your biceps growing as you do a dumbbell curl, or your stomach flattening as you do crunches.

Index